Evaluating the Processes of Neonatal Intensive Care

Thinking Upstream to Im

D1354609

University of
Chester

Evaluating the Processes of Neonatal Intensive Care

Thinking Upstream to Improve Downstream Outcomes

Joseph Schulman

Associate Professor of Pediatrics, Albany Medical College; and Senior Scientist, Clinical Informatics and Outcomes Research, Children's Hospital at Albany Medical Center, Albany, New York

© BMJ Publishing Group 2004
BMJ Books is an imprint of the BMJ Publishing Group

All rights reserved. No part of this publication may be reproduced,
stored in a retrieval system, or transmitted, in any form or by any
means, electronic, mechanical, photocopying, recording and/or
otherwise, without the prior written permission of the publishers.

First published in 2004
by BMJ Books, BMA House, Tavistock Square,
London WC1H 9JR

www.bmjbooks.com

British Library Cataloguing in Publication Data

A catalogue record for this book is available from the British Library

ISBN 0 7279 1833 8

Typeset by SIVA Math Setters, Chennai, India
Printed and bound in Spain by GraphyCems, Navarra

Contents

In a time of drastic change, it is the learners who inherit the future. The learned find themselves equipped to live in a world that no longer exists.

Eric J Hoffer

Preface

Instead of seeking new landscapes, develop new eyes.

Marcel Proust

Daily, we must justify – explicitly, objectively – what we do in the neonatal intensive care unit (NICU). And increasingly, we must demonstrate that these activities provide value for those we serve and for the money spent. Even the process of accrediting our care facilities now demands that we understand the fine structure of our work, our results, and how these are related. Accreditation will demand too, that we show continual improvement in what we achieve (Joint Commission on Accreditation of Healthcare Organizations ORYX initiative; http://www.jcaho.org/perfmeas/oryx/oryx_frm.htm). If only the skills we acquired during our education and work careers could prove sufficient for meeting these expectations; but all too often our skills fall short of these challenges.[1-4]

For those of us who must close this gap – between our current skill set and the challenges before us – this book aims to send you well along the path toward competently evaluating and improving the work and results of the NICU. I know that you already have too little time in your day. I have strived to make the ideas clear, definite, and relevant; the writing accessible, coherent, and transparent; the conceptual development manageably incremental, intuitive, and logical.

So much of our work, though we look straight at it, lies there unappreciated – important causal relationships remaining obscure unless we specifically think about them and know how to see them. Imagine this: you awaken in a campsite 9000 feet above sea level. The sun is a small orange disc offering no heat, rising above the irregular horizon behind you. The air is frigid, making all you see exist in icy contrast. "I must get a picture of this place," you say to yourself. As you look at the image of a mountain peak through the lens of your camera, you envision a striking photograph. Patches of white snow are carved into jagged shapes by jet-black shadows. In the foreground, outlined by the ethereal yet deep blue sky, lies a palette of colors created by the sunlight filtering through the thin air and impacting the hard slope. Pressing the shutter release, you know you will be proud of the result.

What have you just done in this scenario? "I've taken a picture of a mountain," you might say. Ansel Adams, the noted photographer, might answer differently. He might say you have carefully selected light and thoughtfully captured its effects on the film in your camera. This formulation distinguishes the product from the steps that comprise the production process.

To the extent that we are aware of the component activities of our work, we can then influence or control them.

- We may not think about the component activities at all.
- We may only think about them abstractly. This approach may paradoxically block our inquiry because of the vagueness inherent to abstraction.
- We may actively think about the fine structure of the component activities.

If you are reading this, your daily work probably is associated with a newborn intensive care unit. How do you view your work? Please take a moment to express your thoughts. Perhaps you say something like "My daily work is helping sick infants get better." No doubt, this is what you want to *accomplish* by your work. This is the view that equates taking a picture of a mountain with releasing the camera shutter. In this view, many aspects of achieving the desired result fly by so quickly that they probably go unnoticed. How do we formulate a blur? Our distinguishing what we want to accomplish from what we actually *do* enables greater mastery of our work and a deeper sense of meaning for our profession.

We may consider what we want to accomplish by the activity of the NICU to be the aim of our system of care. What we do to achieve the aim is our work. We implement, coordinate, and interpret the results of a rather complex web of *processes*. The picture-taking scenario included the processes of composing an image, focusing the camera, determining exposure settings, and releasing the shutter. The picture is the *result*. It is an underlying assumption in this book that when we broadly and deeply understand component processes, we get better results.

A few years ago I awoke to the importance of answering the question: How can a neonatology group practice add value to its hospital system? When I discussed this with colleagues, too often the responses resembled: "Well, clearly, we're the quality group," or, "Just look at our outcomes." Amazingly, I never heard anyone express concern that their unit might *not* be as good as another NICU in town.

What do we mean by "a good NICU," or by "doing well?" What are the components of a NICU that add value to the system of hospital care? Answers emerge from examining the fine structure of our work, the results of that work, and considering explicitly why we do our work and how all these concepts are related. For some of us, such a view of clinical neonatology amounts to seeing the NICU with new eyes; and when we do, the landscape changes forever.

We are accustomed to looking at, and thinking mainly about, the end-results of the work of the NICU. "End-results" ordinarily is a redundant word pair. But in this book the term discriminates between terminal and intermediary process results. Often we neglect to examine how the results occurred or how we might alter what we do so that we may get different results.[5] This book is an invitation to look at and think about what goes on "upstream," in our care processes, so that we may understand and influence the causal webs producing what some call outcomes – the "downstream" end-results.

References

1 Horbar JD. *A national evidence-based quality improvement collaborative for neonatology, Vermont Oxford Network, 1997, Annual Network Update.* Washington, DC, December 7, 1997.
2 Horbar JD. Personal communication based on data from NICUs participating in the Vermont Oxford Clinical Trials Network. Burlington, VT, April 20, 1998.
3 Horbar JD. The Vermont Oxford Network: evidence-based quality improvement for neonatology. *Pediatrics* 1999;**103**(1 suppl E):350–9.
4 McCormick MC. Quality of care: an overdue agenda. *Pediatrics* 1997;**99**:249–50.
5 McCormick MC. The outcomes of very low birth weight infants: are we asking the right questions? *Pediatrics* 1997;**99**:869–76.

Introduction

Given the importance of health care, it seems inconceivable that we do not have excellent ways of evaluating how well we are doing. Yet the fact is, we do not ... substandard performance is largely invisible except through a statistical lens.

David M Eddy (1998)[1]

We don't work alone

I glance at a pencil resting on my desk and I wonder: Is anyone on this planet sufficiently knowledgeable to make a pencil? This apparently simple tool is the outcome of a complex production system involving many people applying diverse knowledge. A pencil results from knowledge and action in the fields of forestry, logging, wood curing, making graphite, making tools, making fuel ... and so on. The various roles of the many people involved in making the pencil must be carefully coordinated so that it eventually comes to rest on my desk.

The situation is the same in the NICU. No single person saves a baby. Because of many people doing many things in coordination, an infant, at one time desperately ill, eventually leaves the unit in his or her mother's arms.

Work standards

Now consider your one job among the many in the NICU. Think for a moment how you decide that you do your job well. How do you know you did the best possible for that infant going home with their mother? How do you know you did the best possible for the unfortunate infant who did not recover? Do you have explicit standards? If you do have standards for judging your work, how did you get them? Or is it just obvious that you are a good doctor, a good nurse? If you had to, could you prove it? How?

Three core questions

This book prepares you to judge and to improve your work and the results of your work. We develop clearly expressed and reasonably sequenced ideas, aiming to answer three fundamental questions:

1 How are we doing?
2 How do we know?
3 How can we do better?

Trying to answer these questions keeps you engaged with your work. This effort continually poses new challenges, and by accepting them you will force incremental growth in your skills. Combined with work aims that you believe in, this is the basis of meaningful and gratifying work.[2]

Probing the variation among providers; "drilling down" in our work

Wherever and whenever investigators look at the work of health care, they always find variation in what is done.[3–6] Practice variation, often unrelated to outcome, is causing physicians to lose control in their clinical activities. They are losing control because this variation undermines their scientific legitimacy.[4] Key organizations are questioning whether physicians really know how to evaluate what they do or know how to improve it.[4] Some claim that variation is desirable – it is basic to the art of medicine. This position is indefensible until we can describe and understand the causes and the consequences of the variation (and currently we can't).

To characterize and understand the causes and the consequences of variation in neonatal care we must first understand the daily work of the NICU. Recall the discussion at the beginning of this chapter about the pencil. We seek a broad perspective of work, one that encompasses the *entire* set of tasks involved in NICU operation. Although some readers may have experience examining the more evidently important tasks, the total number of tasks is large, and we have yet to understand them in aggregate. Many of the tasks may seem mundane and uninviting of scrutiny. Until we carefully examine and understand them all, singly and in their relation to each other, any ranking by relative importance may be wrong. Wrong too, may be our proposed remedies for problems.

To consider seriously the entire set of processes comprising the NICU is intellectually stimulating and can yield profound insights for improving the results of neonatal care. But remember that a few days of continuing medical education may not undo years of professional habits. (Think about this point too when you read Chapter 1, "Systems and our work.") Habits are usually difficult to change because often they are not isolated behaviors; rather, they are enmeshed with *many* aspects of the systems of which they are a part. Overcoming the difficulty with such change may relate to understanding and working with those interconnections. So take the material in this book and reiteratively think about it, relate it to your experience, struggle with it; *make it part of your daily work, make it part of the way you think.* Do these things from many perspectives, so the interconnections that tend to make old habits hard to eradicate become evident; and once so, the habits are not needed – indeed, not wanted. Along the way you will likely discover new enjoyment of your work.

What is quality?

Sooner or later, discussions about improving the care in the NICU touch on the notion of quality. Let's take care of it sooner. How do you define quality? That which emerges when the most resources available are brought to bear on a problem? That which emerges when the most skilled people are involved in a process? Might it simply be whatever a patient (parent) says it is? Perhaps quality is what a consumer buys for the dollars spent in the NICU. In this context, some people believe we should know which NICUs provide better value for money.

Now consider the consensus statement by The Institute of Medicine (IOM) National Roundtable on Health Care Quality:

The quality of health care can be precisely defined and measured with a degree of scientific accuracy comparable with that of most measures used in clinical medicine. Serious and widespread quality problems exist throughout American medicine. These problems, which may be classified as overuse, underuse, and misuse, occur in small and large communities alike, in all parts of the country, and with approximately equal frequency in managed care and fee-for-service systems of care. Very large numbers of Americans are harmed as a direct result. Quality of care is the problem, not managed care. Current efforts to improve will not succeed unless we undertake a major, systematic effort to overhaul how we deliver health care services, educate and train clinicians, and assess and improve quality.[7]

If you merely scanned this paragraph in small print, please go back and read it slowly. The powerful statements, well documented in the report, clearly call for reconsidering old beliefs, and changing what we do. Precisely how does the IOM define the notion of quality?

The IOM calls quality of care:

... the degree to which health services for individuals and populations increase the likelihood of desired health outcomes and are consistent with current professional knowledge.[7]

For many years now, this definition has withstood critical review from various perspectives and remains useful. It is robust. Here again, I suggest a second reading. Notice that it implies a causal relationship between health services and health outcomes. Recall this definition of quality as you engage with the entire set of tasks involved in neonatal care, and as you measure causal events and end-results.

How we will approach quality improvement?

This book aims to help improve the mean level of quality (using the operational definition of the IOM) in your NICU. We will take a systems perspective, to explore how the systems we create allow or even facilitate errors and waste. We will eschew an all too common habit of blaming individuals for errors when all they were doing was what the system demanded of them. We will examine processes and outcomes, indicating the importance and need for process data and showing limitations of some outcome data. "Process data are usually more sensitive measures of quality than outcome data, because a poor outcome does not occur every time there is an error in the provision of care."[8]

Lessons from Japan about quality and cost

In 1984 the infant mortality rate in Japan was one half that in the United States (US). Perhaps even more surprising, Japan's per capita spending on health care was one third that of the US. Remarkably, the English language health care literature and the Ministry of Health in Tokyo offered no comprehensive explanation for the phenomenon. Japanese auto manufacturers were then a focus of attention in the US, and my hunch was that the efficiency of the Japanese health care system was a reflection of a Toyota-like approach to delivering health care. In 1986 I obtained support from the World Health Organization (WHO) and the US Department of Health, Education, and Welfare (HEW) to learn about delivery and outcomes (including cost) of health care for infants in Japan.

Surely, I thought, such good health outcomes at such relatively low cost must reflect an advanced production process. This was correct, but not primarily with respect to the hospital-based neonatal health care process. I learned that the advanced production process (resulting in low infant mortality rates) was based more in the cultural norms of everyday life rather than in the organizations directly delivering health care. The Japanese way of living appeared to produce healthier babies.[9] Societal resources seemed more devoted to *preventing* problems than *fixing* them after they occurred. As a result, demand for the more expensive component of the infant health care system – newborn intensive care – was low, and so was total resource use for neonatal care. Further, low demand sectors understandably experienced little pressure to become organizationally advanced. Today the health care systems of many countries are under pressure to develop advanced and more efficient methods. Per capita spending on health care in the United States (US) exceeded 14% of GDP by 1993 (data from Organization for Economic Cooperation and Development (OECD), 1995[10]), remained approximately level for the decade, and is projected to exceed 16% of GDP by the end of 2010 (Centers for Medicare and Medicaid Services[11]).

Regrettably, I did not visit the production facilities of Toyota during my work in Japan. This company has successfully inverted the relationship between quality and cost that originally obtained in the automobile industry. No longer do economists maintain that as quality improves cost must increase. Toyota accomplished the inverse relation between quality and cost by changing from mass production to "lean production," and their methods are applicable to perhaps all areas of human activity.[12]

Lean production combines aspects of craft production and mass production. Craft production entails highly skilled workers making a particular thing that a client commissions. The craftsperson and the client are usually pleased with the work and the results, but the process is expensive. Mass production was developed early in this century in an attempt to bring goods to more people at lower cost. Mass production turns out a large number of standard products at relatively low cost. In this case, workers often complain of unfulfilling work conditions while the consumer, given the choice, often seems to prefer a version produced by a craftsperson (better quality).

Why, you may ask, do we seem to digress and now discuss producing cars? We do so because factors that turned around the fortunes of Toyota after World War II illuminate important premises in our story about evaluating and improving neonatal care.

Lean production is a way of making things that involves continuous improvement. Lean production is "lean" because more product results from fewer resources. Mass producers and lean producers think differently about their products. Mass producers set quality standards at "good enough." It would just be too expensive to do better. *Their quality focus is downstream, on the end results.* They inspect what appears at the end of the production line and make final adjustments by reworking the end result. *For lean producers, on the other hand, the focus is rather diffuse – they look upstream and downstream.* They alter end results by adjusting upstream processes, *preventing* the problems that mass producers discover during final inspection. Lean producers are after perfection. They know this goal is unreachable, but using it as the standard underlies their success. Aiming for perfection changes the way people work, the way they think, and (yes), even the way they live.[12]

A view of the work of the NICU

Perhaps you haven't thought of it this way before, but we make things in the NICU. The NICU is truly a production facility. And we have much to learn from the experience of others working with the problems of producing things. Clarifying our understanding of what we make, why we make it, and how we can make it better, can improve NICU outcomes. In later chapters we will talk about a variety of outcomes. For now, we can broadly categorize NICU outcomes as patient end-results and resources used.

Improving end-results for patients is a tenet of medical professionalism. For some professionals, concern for the resources used in achieving the patient end-results may seem irrelevant or even unethical. I believe such attitudes reflect incomplete understanding of the aims of an individual NICU (we will expand upon the notion of aims in a little while). Indeed, many parallels may be drawn between the perspectives of American automobile manufacturers during the 1970s particularly, and the perspectives of many health care professionals trained during or before the same period.

When we deny the need to continually adapt to a changing environment, to changing inputs, and to changing customer expectations, we open a niche for a shrewd competitor. The niche would not be there to fill if the changes in the environment were not real. The American automobile manufacturers took a long time to recognize this, but they eventually did. It now seems that American health care professionals are experiencing pressure to alter their world view. We can deny that costs must decrease and patient results and satisfaction levels must improve. Yes, we can deny it, but because the once-protected market status of health care no longer exists, I think the changes in results and cost will happen anyway. Who among us will embrace these changes? Who will lead? And what will the outcomes be like? Thinking about these questions, we may be aided by Toyota's operational insight. Toyota discovered fundamentally not the knowledge for making cars; they discovered the underlying knowledge for making *things*.[12] And we will examine some of this knowledge as it applies to our work in the NICU.

The plan of this book

When the only tool you have is a hammer, everything looks like a nail.

Abraham Maslow

This book provides a useful assortment of tools for varied problem solving but it is not a tool manual. The emphasis is on identifying a problem, understanding its antecedents and effects, and changing those factors and relationships to achieve more desirable results. The tools assist these processes.

We can decide something is a nail because we only have a hammer, or we can decide that something is a nail because definite ways of thinking – decision rules – brought us to that conclusion. In the latter case, having independently determined that, yes, we are dealing with a nail we are then pleased to find we have a hammer in our tool case. This is the approach offered here.

The broad areas we examine are:

1 Systems
2 Activity without value (*Muda*)
3 Tools for understanding systems
4 Identifying and measuring variables
5 Variation in our measurements
6 Benchmarking
7 Keeping track of our evaluative work with an instrument panel display of collected data
8 Leadership and change.

The subject matter is practical – providing multifaceted insight and skills for turning ideas into action. The ways of thinking, methods, and tools reflect the content of a special series of articles, *Quality of Health Care*, published in the *New England Journal of Medicine* in the fall of 1996 (see particularly Chassin[13] and Blumenthal[14]).

Credit for good ideas appearing in this guide belongs to the original thinkers whose work I cite and to the superb faculty at the Center for the Evaluative Clinical Sciences, Dartmouth Medical School, from whom I was privileged to learn during a sabbatical year in Hanover, New Hampshire. My task centers on applying those ideas to what we do in the NICU. The responsibility for the framing and presenting is mine.

My commitment to you

I wish that we could be interacting in person. I am convinced that dialogue, personalized challenges to your thinking, and individualized rephrasing and reiterating are important aspects of creating new mental space for these ideas and skills. I care deeply about effectively communicating with you. I also know that we can learn a great deal from each other.

This project is my greatest work priority and I take the same approach to the work of writing this book as I propose that we do for our work in the NICU. Please don't just read this. Contribute to your own understanding of surveying those you serve, and to my understanding of how to serve you and further readers by sending me your questions, disagreements, elaborations, omissions, improvement suggestions ... anything appropriate. I am also available for on-site consultative support. You can contact me by email at: **schulmj@mail.amc.edu**. Now let's begin transforming our work.

References

1 Eddy DM. Performance measurement: problems and solutions. *Health Affairs* 1998;**17**:7–25.
2 Csikszentmihalyi M. *Finding flow*. New York: Basic Books, 1997.
3 Horbar JD. Personal communication based on data from NICUs participating in the Vermont Oxford Clinical Trials Network. Burlington, VT, April 20, 1998.
4 Blumenthal D. The variation phenomenon in 1994. *N Engl J Med* 1994;**331**:1017–18.
5 Horbar JD, Badger GJ, Lewit EM, *et al.* Hospital and patient characteristics associated with variation in 28-day mortality rates for very low birth weight infants. *Pediatrics* 1997;**99**:149–56.
6 Wennberg JE, ed. The Center for the Evaluative Clinical Sciences, DMS. *The Dartmouth atlas of health care in the United States*. Chicago, IL: American Hospital Publishing, 1998.
7 Chassin MR, Galvin RW, National Roundtable on Health Care Quality. The urgent need to improve health care quality. *JAMA* 1998;**280**:1000–5.
8 Brook RH, McGlynn EA, Cleary PD. Measuring quality of care. *N Engl J Med* 1996;**335**:966–70.
9 Schulman J. Japan's healthy babies – an American doctor's view. *World Health Forum* 1989;**10**:66–9.

10   Folland S, Goodman AC, Stano M. *The economics of health and health care.* Upper Saddle River, NJ: Prentice Hall, 1997.
11   Centers for Medicare and Medicaid Services. *An Overview of the U.S. Healthcare System: Two decades of change, 1980–2000.* http://www.cms. hhs.gov/charts/healthcaresystem/chapter1.pdf (accessed 15 Dec 2003).
12   Womack JP, Jones DT, Roos D. *The machine that changed the world: the story of lean production.* New York: HarperCollins, 1990.
13   Chassin MR. Improving the quality of care. *N Engl J Med* 1996;**335**: 1060–3.
14   Blumenthal D. The origins of the quality-of-care debate. *N Engl J Med* 1996;**335**:1146–9.

Part 1:
Systems

Every system is perfectly designed to achieve the results that it gets.

Paul B Batalden and Donald M Berwick attribute
this insight to each other

1: Systems and our work

Practical sciences proceed by building up; theoretical sciences by resolving into components.

[Saint] Thomas Aquinas (ca. 1225–1274)

Our usual way of thinking (typical, linear thinking)

Sometimes we approach a problem by *analyzing* it; we take it apart. This approach is common in Western cultures, and in some scientific disciplines. We often think in terms of linear relationships among the parts. The linear problem-solving paradigm entails identifying a cause for an effect of interest. Unfortunately, it works better for getting good grades on academic examinations than for solving the complex and messy problems of the real world.

Thinking about interrelationships

Alternatively, we can approach a problem by *synthesizing*; we look at the greater context in which the problem exists. We look for interrelationships among the parts of the relevant causal system. But we do not focus on one part of the system; we try to consider the whole. This is difficult. Often the systems we work with are terribly complex, so this approach can overwhelm our thinking abilities. (Later, we will also discuss how an individual cause, *external* to the system, may be related to an effect on system performance.)

The easy and convenient way out of the difficulty is to simply avoid this way of thinking. Systems thinkers believe that such dodging facilitates problems coming back after they've been "solved." That is, they were "solved" analytically when they should have been approached synthetically, systemically. We will return to this point later in this chapter.

Most people spend more time and energy going around problems than in trying to solve them.

Henry Ford

We don't see things as they are, we see things as we are.

Anaïs Nin

Operational definitions

A group ensures that each member thinks about and measures one and the same thing by operationally defining it. This introduces clarity and precision to a concept and minimizes inter-observer variation. In general, a definition assigns an object to a class and describes the unique identifying characteristics for that object within the class. For example, mortality rate (here, mortality rate is the object to be defined) is a death measure (this is the class assignment) expressing the number of deaths among a specified population of individuals during a specified period of time. Case fatality rate also belongs to the class of death measures, but here the numerator counts deaths from a specific disease and the denominator includes the number of cases of a particular disease among a specified population during a specified period of time. By explicitly stating the criteria and tests that we use to uniquely identify our measurement variable, we allow all individuals reviewing the results to come to the same conclusion. Otherwise, we miss the forest for the trees and cannot even agree on how many trees there are.

Systems

No man is an island entire of itself; every man is ... a part of the main ... any man's death diminishes me because I am involved in Mankind; And therefore never send to know for whom the bell tolls; It tolls for thee.

John Donne

A system is a discrete entity whose function is determined by its interacting component parts. Of course, we are familiar with biological systems, especially human ones. We also are familiar with systems created by people – for example: cars, computers, governments, hospitals, NICUs. The parts of a system and how they interact determine what a system does. A system part is not autonomously functional. For example, your eyes do not see, you (the system) do; a mechanical ventilator does not autonomously ventilate an infant – the NICU system mechanically ventilates an infant. Decomposing a system does not reveal its essence – what it is about, its aim. What is essential about a system appears only when the system as a whole is working.

We need not understand a system to use it and benefit from it. This point is important. Thus, I don't understand the software code for the word processing program I am presently writing with. (Some might consider this an example of a system within a system: a software program operating within a computer; another example: an NICU operating within a hospital.) Yet I believe that I am competently using the program to produce this manuscript. Might some of us confuse the ability to function competently in an NICU with a deep understanding of the NICU as a system?

System aims

At least for systems created by people, a system has a purpose, an aim. The aim of an NICU clarifies for the workers and for the outside world why it exists, why it does what it does. A well-defined aim also sets boundaries for what the system does, and at least implicitly addresses what it does not do. Thinking about the following three questions can clarify NICU aims and operation:[1]

1 Why do we provide the service that we do?
2 How do we provide the service that we do?
3 How do we improve the service?

What are the aims of your NICU? Take a moment right now and try creating a statement of the aims of your unit. The task may seem trivial and you might think that the results are self-evident, until you actually try it. Clearly stating the aims of your NICU is difficult but useful work – it is a prerequisite for coherent improvement.

Explicit aims that reflect the capabilities of the NICU and the benefits to its patients will serve as guideposts for the daily decisions regarding care and the higher level decisions for planning and management of the unit. However, too much specificity about implementing the service can restrict innovation and improvement. For example, a carriage shop of the early 1900s that identified its aim as making a certain type of horse-drawn carriage faced a different future from a shop with an aim to produce transportation conveyances for people. (This observation is adapted from one made by Peter Scholtes[2]) The point is to penetrate to the core of the activity and identify the service capabilities rather than the particulars of implementing those capabilities.

As you create your statement of aims for the NICU, try to distinguish between positive and negative goals. A negative goal describes what you don't want to happen. Since these are non-events, negative goals create problems in establishing causal relationships and measuring such things. We may discover many obstacles in trying to attribute non-causality of a rare event to a system or process. We do better to frame goals positively, in terms of the occurrence of a desired event. Such events may be "upstream" predictors of non-events, but now they are positively framed. The point in any case: we want to establish operational definitions for whatever it is we want to measure, allowing unambiguous measurement, so that we can then evaluate it.

How do we know we are meeting our aims?

Think about establishing clear criteria for deciding whether your NICU is achieving its aims. This will amount to an operational definition of how your unit is doing. (This business of operational definitions can get complicated because of nesting, like the Russian dolls that seem to endlessly contain smaller ones within.) Beware of aims that actually rely on implicit precedent goals. For example, consider an aim of preventing neurological injury following cardiopulmonary resuscitation on a neonate. This is an operationally undefined (first problem), negative goal (second problem). It relies on precedent, or "upstream," outcomes – positive goals. In other words, preventing neurological injury is a function of actually achieving certain physiologic outcomes (positive goals) that characterize satisfactory cardiopulmonary performance during resuscitation (and which happen to be inversely related to neurological injury).

As you work on your statement of NICU aims, consider that different people in the system may have varying viewpoints. The viewpoint of the physician commonly appears to have priority, perhaps justified by this person's breadth of professional knowledge. This is wrong. Why does the system exist? What is the aim of the NICU? Do we establish NICUs for physicians or for patients and their families? The center of our universe is the infant and the parents.

System optimization: don't mistake a part for the whole

The best is the enemy of the good.

Voltaire

Optimizing a part detracts from the functioning of the whole. Because of the numerous interrelationships between system components (indicated by the arrows in Figure 1.1), optimizing a part destructively interferes with the intended interactions. Optimizing a part means shifting away from the system aim and adopting a new "aim," focused on the part. This new focus does not resonate with the overarching system aim. For example, the structure and function of the brain reflects the other organs that it interacts with and the assumed goal of an environmentally fit human being. Considering the brain as an isolated information-processing unit is not meaningful.

Work as a system

People working together for a common aim may constitute a system. One conceptual model for work as a system is

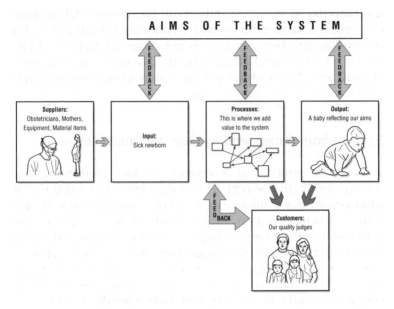

Figure 1.1 A SIPOC model of the NICU

referred to by the acronym SIPOC: Suppliers, Input, Processes, Output and Customers.

Figure 1.1 attempts to illustrate the work of the NICU. It simplifies a very messy and complicated system. "Messy" is not meant to imply unclean or unkempt. I want to connote complex, sometimes untraceable, non-linear interactions and interdependence among system parts. I am referring to relationships so complicated that, even if we succeed in disentangling the components, we are unsure about how to understand what remains. That is what I mean by "messy".

Interrelationships within a system

We may be accustomed to focusing on the boxes and the pictures when we look at charts that describe relationships among things. The boxes and the pictures usually receive names; these diagram elements seem to represent the substantial part of the graphic. Well, there is another part of these diagrams that is at least as important. We denote relationships on these diagrams with arrows. Arrows are crucial parts of a system diagram because systems are about interrelationships. So don't let the small amount of ink devoted to these arrows mislead you. If you don't pay attention to the arrows you'll miss the point. (I couldn't resist.)

System boundaries and system perspectives

Trying to understand a system includes identifying the boundaries of that system. The system boundaries determine what constitutes a subjective or an objective assessment of a system. A subjective perspective simply means we are looking at the system from within. In distinction to believing that the only subjective perspective is our own, note that organizations can yield as many subjective assessments of themselves as the number of their component individuals. An objective perspective looks in on a system from outside it. Here too, more than one assessment is possible. Although modern culture seems to equate "truth" with "objectivity" – the dictionary describes the objective perspective as arising outside the perceptions of an individual (and subjective perspective based in an individual's perceptions)[3] – total objectivity is meaningless because an observer can never stand completely outside all relevant systems. For our purposes, objectivity or subjectivity of perspective is determined by the system boundaries set by the observer.

These notions can frame how we evaluate our systems and results. We will discuss benchmarks and benchmarking in Chapter 11. For now, we may consider judging our NICUs by internal benchmarks as subjective assessment and by external benchmarks as objective assessment.

Can you specify the precise boundaries of your NICU? Are the boundaries truly set by doors and walls? Some NICU processes extend into, and become enmeshed in the processes of other areas of the hospital, and even the community. Think, for example of how your unit interacts with the hospital laboratory, the radiology department, community support services, and visiting nurse services. Indeed, specifying precise boundaries may lead to endless detail, illustrated by trying to determine the precise distance around the island of Great Britain. On a map, there is no problem, but if you try to do it by walking around the island itself, the distance and the difficulty increases with the level of measurement precision.

Key ideas about systems from Senge's rules of the "fifth discipline"

The "fifth discipline" is Peter Senge's term for systems thinking (and the title of his well-known book).[4] Drawn from his formulation, I offer the following observations for understanding the work in the NICU as well as other systems.

1 Sometimes we make a problem "go away" by merely removing it from our direct experience, but not from the system as a whole. This leads to the "push-down/pop-up" effect. Have you ever tried to get rid of a bump on a rug by stepping on it, only to discover the bump re-appears somewhere else on the rug?

2 System components can respond to your intervention and compensate for the changes you make. When this happens, rather than ratchet-up our efforts ("We're not easily beaten – we'll just work twice as hard!") consider a higher order solution – a sweeping, qualitative change that changes the system itself.

3 The compensating response a system makes to your intervention may take months or years to appear. By then, much may have changed, including the staff. Recognizing that a "new" problem is actually the delayed response to a change implemented a long time ago may be a nearly impossible intellectual feat. Many other changes likely occurred in the interim. Which, if any are causally related? So whenever possible, don't do many things at once – the effects may be uninterpretable.

4 The most obvious problem or the one that we have special competence to solve is not necessarily the most important one. Similarly, beware of making the problem conform to your skills rather than the other way around. (Recall Maslow's aphorism in the Introduction about the hammer and the nail.)

5   Sometimes a short-term improvement may create a long-term dependency. Examples abound among government programs. Consider how much of our work in the NICU may be related to governmental policy on income distribution, education, access to care, or to reimbursement mechanisms.

6   If you accept the premise that understanding complex systems can test the limits of human thinking, then consider the likelihood of rapid organizational growth or change producing desirable long-term results. This situation should not justify inaction. Rather, the observation emphasizes the need for well-informed and well-reasoned action.

7   A cause can be, and often is, a complex interaction of factors (multiple causation). Similarly, an effect may be a manifestation of complex interactions.

8   "Leverage" is the term describing the significant effect of a seemingly small, but precisely directed intervention on a system. Often, the areas of highest leverage are initially obscure. They become apparent with detailed study of the system. In other words, the solution to a problem offered "off the top of one's head" often turns out not to be the one with greatest beneficial effect. Are such solutions rarely put forth in hospitals?

9   Remember the importance of the time dimension. In this book we will frequently refer to the time dimension, particularly when we discuss measurement and variation. System "snapshots" are inaccurate by at least one dimension. Drawing inferences about dynamic performance from a static assessment risks erroneous conclusions.

10 "Dividing an elephant in half does not produce two small elephants."[4] If you understand the definition of a system, then you appreciate the problems associated with organizational "downsizing." Further, the leverage points for the desired change may reside in the amputated portion of the system.

11 Blaming an individual for a problem localized to his part of the system is often inaccurate and wrong. The blamee and the blamer are part of the same system. The system drives behavior: objectionable behavior is often a manifestation of system structure and function. Typically,

the blamee was merely doing what the system required. Because of the interconnectedness in a system, pointing a finger of blame will often eventually result in pointing at most people in the system, including you.

The results are produced by the system. If you don't like the results, work with the system (we examine this notion in particular detail in Chapter 9).

Reconciling a single, isolated cause with systems thinking

Sometimes, rather than implicate a complex causal web we are able to identify one discrete cause for a problem. Finding a single, isolated cause residing within a system is unusual. Instead, a single cause may be identified to originate outside the system, although it may affect many interrelated system components. Neonatal infection with group B streptococcus is an example.

How are we to understand the effects of single causes on multifactorial webs (systems)? The answer lies in the concepts relating to understanding variation, a topic we examine in Chapter 9. These extra-systemic single causes are so-called *external* perturbations to an otherwise stable system. We refer to these external perturbations as "special causes" of variation.

References

1 Langley GJ, Nolan KM, Nolan TW, *et al. The improvement guide.* San Francisco: Jossey-Bass, 1996.
2 Scholtes PR. *The leader's handbook.* New York: McGraw-Hill, 1998.
3 Mish FC, ed. *Merriam-Webster's collegiate dictionary.* Springfield, MA: Merriam-Webster, Inc., 1993.
4 Senge PM. *The fifth discipline.* New York: Doubleday, 1990.

2: The work of the NICU

Processes: general understanding

The processes of a system convert inputs to outputs. Processes are not capable on their own of achieving the aims of the overall system. When processes become complex and relate to other processes, the distinction from a system gets fuzzy, like the distinction between a boat and a ship. A process is composed of methods – appreciated only in the context of the process. Methods are composed of steps. Think of steps as the basic events that in aggregate become a method. For example:

- System – a hospital
- System, but less well bounded – NICU
- Process – making rounds
- Method – starting with the patient at the northeast corner of the NICU, proceeding sequentially, comprehensively reviewing patient data available since the last review
- Step – going to radiology and seeing all recent films.

These distinctions are quite useful for conceptualizing work. And as writing is to thinking, so *process mapping* is to conceptualizing work. A process map is a detailed flow chart depicting the components of our processes. A process map clarifies our methods and steps as we conceptually "drill down" into our daily activities and make explicit these components that otherwise often are unapparent.

As shown by Figure 1.1 in Chapter 1, individual processes may be linked to one another. For example: conducting morning rounds, the pharmacy preparing the day's TPN orders, the laboratory running the previously ordered morning chemistry and hematology tests, and the obstetricians performing three consecutive C-sections requiring the neonatologist's attendance, are all linked, interacting processes.

Processes: getting to the core of the work

When we comprehensively map the processes of our work, we discover that some of the linked processes are conceptually associated in a "core" representing the basic work of the system.[1] Other processes represent supportive linkages. This distinction is not made for the sake of further hierarchical organization; rather, it assists with prioritizing among the activities. The Japanese consider this approach so helpful they have a special word for it, *Gemba*. Interestingly, we have no similar word in English. Roughly, it means the collection of things we directly use and do for adding value to the object of our processes. Thus, intubating an infant in respiratory failure is *Gemba*; waiting in the surgical lounge for a C-section to occur is not.

Process mapping

Here are some tips for process mapping.[1]

- Just as you rearrange paragraphs to achieve coherence in a piece of writing, process mapping involves lots of rearranging of steps and methods before settling on a depiction of reality. Writing the component names on Post-it Notes facilitates moving the ideas around on a display board.
- Start by naming the processes in the system. Use one process per Post-it Note. Remember that a process is an activity, the "doing" of something, so to stay consistent in your thinking, use names ending with the suffix: "-ing." NICU examples include admitting, feeding, prescribing, intubating, and ventilating.
- Distinguish the core work processes, the *Gemba*, and the support processes enabling the *Gemba*. You might try different color Post-it Notes to set off *Gemba* from support. "Supportive processes that do not 'know' the core process steps they support and that do not 'know' how they provide support are common examples of suboptimization."[1]
- Arrange the processes to reflect what actually happens (most of the time) to an infant receiving care in the NICU. Describe what is, not what you would like to see. That is the only way to improve the current reality.
- The more people *from* the process that are *doing the mapping*, the more the map will reflect reality.

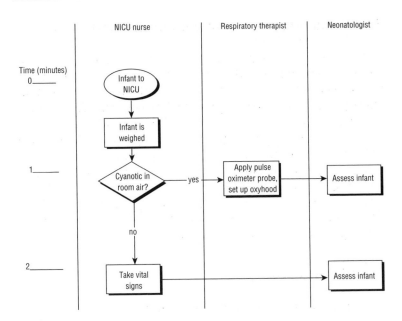

Figure 2.1 A deployment chart mapping the early steps of admitting an infant to the NICU

Process mapping is a prerequisite for meaningful system measurement. It clarifies the current reality and uncovers waste in the system. Process maps may have different formats. *The memory jogger II* is a helpful guide to many of the tools we discuss, including process mapping.[2] This little book supplements the overview you find here.

I particularly like the deployment format for process mapping because it depicts how a wide array of multi-dimensional information is associated. One chart can show what happens, in what sequence, by whom, and when. For example, Figure 2.1 shows a small portion of the admitting process.

Further tips for process mapping.[1]

- By creating a deployment chart you may discover that currently no one "owns" a process or step.
- Look for recursive loops – a sign that a process area may not be adding value.
- Identify explicitly the starting and finishing steps. For example, "The process of admitting a neonate to the unit

begins when .... (fill in an individual role) does .... "
(fill in a specific step).

Process mapping is not as difficult as genome mapping, but
if you've never tried it prepare for a challenging and time-
consuming activity that is well worth the effort.

Analyzing a process map

Consider the following as you study the process map you
have created.[3] Keep a written record of your assessment – it
will inform subsequent improvement efforts.

- For each activity (rectangular symbol) on the chart:

  - Is it redundant?
  - Does it add value? What do you think about the
    relative cost?
  - How does the process prevent errors in this activity?
  - Who "owns" this?
  - Try describing the variation in results and what is
    known about the causes (see the chapters on variation).

- For each decision point (diamond-shaped symbol):

  - Verify that the decision involves a check on what has
    gone before. Is this check an absolute filter for errors?
    Have we already checked the same thing?

- For each place where work is handed off from one person
  to another:

  - Identify who is involved.
  - Identify what could go wrong.

- Looking at the overall flow of work:

  - Does the arrangement of steps make sense?
  - Is our diagram all-inclusive? Can anything get lost "in
    the cracks?"
  - If there is more than one path for something to occur:
    Are the conditions for a particular path explicit and
    appropriate?

- If you diagram a "rework" loop, understand:

- If the process performs without failure, is this rework path needed?
- How much this loop entails (in steps, time, resources, etc.).
- Does proceeding through the loop prevent recurring failure?
- How many sources of information are needed to assess the loop?

- Use customer knowledge and the aim of the system as guideposts for analyzing the process.
- Check your analysis with others involved with the process.

Customers

As you explore the concept of a customer the notion becomes increasingly complex. Here are two definitions.

- The customer is the beneficiary of what we do and make.
- The customer is anyone who can be disappointed or angry over what we do and make.[4] (I particularly like this definition.)

We may also want to distinguish internal and external customers. External customers refer to the traditional notion of the ultimate service recipient. Internal customers are those more deeply embedded in our system. Table 2.1 gives some examples from an NICU perspective.

Because of the complex interrelationships in our systems, we can please or anger many people in the course of doing our work. Our knowing and acting on this demonstrates systems thinking – thinking with an aim to optimize the function of the whole, not just a part.

Whose perspective is most appropriate to guide what is done in the NICU? I think it is arrogant to believe "the doctor, or the NICU team knows best." When you communicate with parents do you persuade or do you enter into a dialog? Reflect a while on how our more laudable professional traits – thoughtfulness ("What else can we do for the infant and her parents?"), empathy, responsiveness, and altruism – can affect

Table 2.1 Type of customer *	
Customer	**Type**
Neonate	External
Parents	External
Medical learners	Internal
Obstetrician	Internal
Hospital administrator	Internal
NICU nurse	Internal
The community we work in	External

the way we configure our care processes. Consider too, in whose perspective we should anchor these traits.

When we apply a systems and a customer perspective to our work in the NICU we also want to verify that, to the extent reasonable, people participating in the system are doing so voluntarily. In other words, "unhappy campers" are a signal that the system hasn't got it right. (Did you first think "blame" at the mention of "unhappy campers?" Recall the observation in Chapter 1 that discussed how the system drives behavior.)

Customer knowledge

Sometimes in the NICU, we forget that a patient or a customer has a life with horizons extending widely in time and space. Recognizing this amplifies our ability to empathize and to care for them.

If we want to please our customers, we must understand at least two aspects of their decision process:

1 How do our customers decide about how *we* are doing in the NICU? What do *they* measure? What are *their* judgment criteria?

2 What is it about our customers that might make them use the approach that they do for assessing quality?

This knowledge greatly facilitates our efforts to improve what we do – importantly, in ways that reflect the needs of those we serve. Most of us know the feeling of surprise when a patient's (parent's) service quality assessment varies with our own view. But do we dismiss the discrepancy because we think the patient (parent) is relatively uninformed, or do we welcome the opportunity for fresh insight about how our work appears to the person the NICU was created to serve? Appearing to care about our customers won't do. The concern must be genuine. Then, our defensive barriers to feedback drop and conduits of customer knowledge open. Listening to those we serve is at the heart of doing a good job.

Here are some conduits through which we may listen to our customers:

- complaints
- questions
- parent support groups
- satisfaction surveys (see next section)
- adverse outcome reports.

Matching the service with the customer need

One useful way to analyze customer satisfaction compares what someone needs with what the system provides.[4] This kind of thinking is related to the concept of waste activity, a subject we consider in another chapter. We can arrange service and need in four ways.

1 The customer gets what she needs.
2 The customer doesn't get what she needs.
3 The customer gets what she doesn't need.
4 The customer doesn't get what she doesn't need.

The list suggests a customer survey approach based on two questions.[4]

- What are you getting that you don't need?
- What do you need that you are not getting?

Simple, but comprehensive.

Table 2.2   Illustrations of NICU inputs

Input category	NICU examples
Human	The patient The neonatologist The nurse
Information	Database The neonatologist's skills, memory The nurse's skills, memory

Material	Epuipment
	   Overhead warmers
	   Isolettes
	   Mechanical ventilators

Financial	Grants Regular budget allowance Contractual reimbursement arrangements

Process inputs

Inputs are the things your processes work with. Inputs can be internal or external to the NICU. When we explicitly identify the inputs, when we understand what enters our system and how these things can vary, we build knowledge of how inputs can influence our processes and results. Table 2.2 provides some illustrations of NICU inputs.

Detailed knowledge of inputs informs benchmarking work (judging performance results – see Chapter 11) and allows fairly comparing NICUs (risk adjusting).[5]

Suppliers

The people, departments, and organizations that provide our inputs represent our suppliers. To understand the work of the NICU we must therefore identify each input component's supplier, along the lines of Table 2.2. Who is our source of patients, of goods and equipment, of personnel? Suppliers can be internal or external to the NICU. Suppliers are not restricted to only that role. For example, a supplier may also be a customer. NICU examples of someone in this dual role include the obstetrician and the mother.

Vision: seeing the bigger picture

Vision, as I use the term here, involves synthesizing. With knowledge of your customers and of your community's need for your NICU, you develop an NICU aim for the future. This is not a corporate style waste of time; it is an important activity. Working on a vision – the aim for your NICU in the future – involves assessing the changes going on around and within your NICU. So framed, vision contributes to preventing future waste activity and maximizing future added value.

The aims of the NICU guide current decisions and activities. The *vision* for the NICU represents the aim of our improvement efforts, guiding what we want to be. Here are some tips for thinking about and working on your vision for your NICU.[1]

- Align your vision with community need and customer knowledge.
- We've already discussed trying to understand how your customers judge the quality of your end-results. Now, think about, and make a list of what it will take for your unit to better please those it serves. Include items that your customers have not thought of, but if provided would delight them. (Are you beginning to see how knowledge of one component of the system informs your understanding of another, how they are complexly interrelated?)
- Earlier I indicated how over-specific aims can restrict the adaptability of a system. Vision statements need to be *more* specific and concrete than statements of aims. You are trying to create a detailed picture of what the NICU will look like in the future. You want an implementable blueprint.
- Ask those you serve to read your vision statement. They should feel it reflects their needs and values. They should be pleased with what you want to do.
- Don't create a vision statement and be done with it. Keep working on it over time, continually updating and bringing the picture into sharper focus.

The improvement plan: identify the performance gaps, look for leverage points, "design and redesign"[1]

Using your knowledge of the NICU as a system – its customers, inputs, processes, and results, and using your vision for the future – your plan for maximizing the value of your service in the future, Batalden and Mohr suggest identifying a few improvement themes for the next one to two years.[1] Our system knowledge and vision for the future define gaps between what is and what we want to be. These gaps drive our improvement plans.

From our process knowledge we look for leverage points to effect system improvement. But we are not yet ready to put our ideas into action. We need to consider more specifically how we identify these leverage points, how we might change their current configurations, and how we evaluate our actions. That is the material of the coming chapters.

Every system is perfectly designed to achieve the results that it gets.

Paul B Batalden and Donald M Berwick
attribute this insight to each other

If you keep doing what you've been doing, you will keep getting what you've been getting. So groups (that is, the NICU staff) must accept responsibility (distinguish this from blame) for aspects of the current reality they want to change.

References

1 Batalden PB, Mohr JJ. Building knowledge of health care as a system. *Quality Management in Health Care* 1997;5:1–12.
2 Brassard M, Ritter D. *The memory jogger II.* Methuen, MA: GOAL/QPC, 1994.
3 Mohr J, Batalden P, Nelson G. *Flowcharting, a guide for depicting a process.* Hanover, NH: Center for the Evaluative Clinical Sciences, Dartmouth Medical School, 1995.
4 Scholtes PR. *The leader's handbook.* New York: McGraw-Hill, 1998.
5 Iezzoni LI, ed. *Risk adjusting for measuring healthcare outcomes.* Chicago: Health Administration Press, 1997.

3: Working with process mapping: an example

A process for identifying and treating acute pneumothorax

A NICU team collected data relating to care for pneumothorax. After reviewing their data, they determined to decrease the time between identifying an acute physiologic change compatible with onset of pneumothorax and securing a functioning thoracostomy tube. They needed process information to understand their results. They mapped the process of nursing assessment for an infant at risk of developing a pneumothorax (see Figure 3.1).

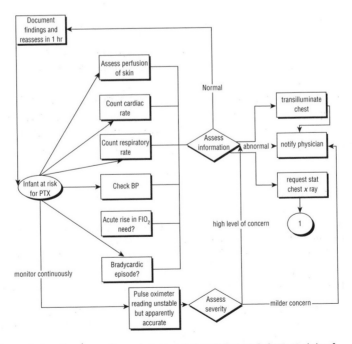

Figure 3.1 Process of nursing assessment for an infant at risk of developing a pneumothorax

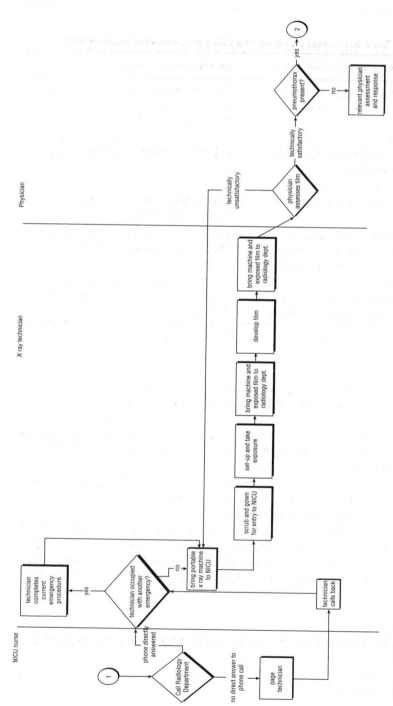

Figure 3.2 Process map for obtaining a chest x ray

Table 3.1   Areas of potential delay and ideas for improvement

Area of potential delay	Idea for improvement*
Contact radiology technician via paging device	Radiology technician to carry cellular phone allowing for direct communication (eliminate a process step)
Technician occupied by another procedure away from NICU	Develop back-up protocol (redesign the process to reflect knowledge of the customer)
Technician brings portable x ray machine to NICU	Keep portable machine immediately outside NICU (combine steps to improve work flow)
Technician returns to radiology department to develop the exposed film	Place a film processing unit in or near NICU (combine steps to improve work flow)
Technician makes return trip to NICU with developed film for neonatologist to read	Place a film processing unit in or near NICU (combine steps to improve work flow)

*Generic change ideas in parentheses reflect material in Chapter 4.

At this first stage of study, the team agreed that moving the procedure of transilluminating a patient's chest to the *initial* screening panel might be a helpful change. They also identified the need for operational definitions of a nursing assessment deemed concerning for the possibility of pneumothorax, as well as for a normal assessment.

They next created a process map for obtaining a stat chest x ray (see Figure 3.2; the circle shape with the number "1" continues from Figure 3.1).

From this map the team identified areas of potential delay, and corresponding ideas for improvement (see Table 3.1). The circle shape with the number "2" inside, at the extreme right of the figure, leads to a map for the process of placing a chest tube in an infant (not presented here).

Further suggestions by NICU staff for improvement

Generic change ideas in parentheses reflect material in Chapter 4.

1 Develop a mutually agreed on method for the radiology department's prioritizing of stat requests (redesign the process to reflect knowledge of the customer).

2 Assign a specific technician on each shift responsibility for the NICU (smooth out handoffs between steps).

3 Develop criteria for bag ventilating a baby when unstable on a ventilator. Note that neither process map refers to this. Because the processes were mapped as they truly were rather than as they should be, the team was able to identify this area of deficiency. Once the team began thinking this way, they recognized the next point below.

4 The team had no explicit process descriptions for the mapped nursing assessments.

5 Develop operational definitions for characterizing the screening assessment by the nurse, as presented in the first map.

If process ownership is not assigned, there may be no real process

On their first review the team had no concerns about the process map for placing a chest tube (not reproduced here), denoted in Figure 3.2 by the circle containing the number "2." When they observed the actual process of placing a chest tube however, (done by a so-called fly-on-the-wall, an uninvolved but meticulous observer), one issue was immediately apparent – lack of process ownership. In the formal mapping exercise, specific duties in specific sequence were assigned to the NICU nurse. But the NICU has more than one nurse. The process as it existed did not assign specific steps to a particular nurse. Observing the actual steps in placing a chest tube from a nursing frame of reference showed *no* process at all. Because one nurse assumed the other had performed them, some tasks were not done; other tasks were needlessly duplicated. The staff clearly saw the need for several people to carry out all necessary steps, but precisely who did what was dangerously ambiguous.

So here is an example of a "process" that appeared fine – but only when the team examined it in a dispassionate exercise that was devoid of the urgency which accompanies the reality they tried to map. When the mapping was performed during that actual urgent event, evidently there was no nursing-level process!

From this exercise, the team came to appreciate deployment process mapping. They learned about what exceedingly specific detailed knowledge they needed to understand the fine structure of their processes. Further, they discovered a new sense of control over their work.

4: Activity without value: *muda*

Activity without value: a systems framing

Much of the evaluative work in the NICU centers on answering two questions:

1 Are we doing the right thing?
2 Are we doing the right thing well?

Of the first, when the answer is affirmative we may say we are *effective*. For example, about a decade ago researchers used clinical trials to evaluate the effectiveness of artificial surfactant. They learned that by using artificial surfactant neonatologists could increase the survival rate of infants desperately ill from surfactant deficiency. The trials informed us that we were doing the right thing to use artificial surfactant in the operationally defined context of the studies.

We are *efficient* when we are doing the right thing *and* we are doing it well. Fine, now we need to operationally define "doing it well." This will not be easy, because each of our processes will need its own operational definition for "doing it well." But consider this: until you define how you know that you are doing well, how can you say you are doing well? As you continue to read, do you feel a progressively greater tug on your professional foundation? Are you beginning to question the basis by which previously you judged your work?

Now, having thus framed effectiveness and efficiency, how shall we consider efforts not closely aligned with these ideas? We may say that such efforts represent activity without value.

Muda and some assumptions about efficiency and waste

The Japanese have a single word for this concept of activity without value: *muda*. How many examples of *muda* in your

NICU system can you think of, right now? I shall guess that your list is not long – we tend to underestimate the proportion of our activity without value. Yes, I am speaking about the work of health professionals, physicians, nurses, and others. After all, if we gave priority to thinking about the pervasiveness and prevalence of waste, I suspect our descriptive vocabulary might contain a richer array of nuance than we find in the dictionary. So let's "drill down" and think about the varied manifestations of *muda*, activity without value.

How vaguely or how clearly we think about *muda* affects our basic views on work, so please consider these questions.[1]

1 Are the keys to greater efficiency and productivity (assume reasonable operational definitions of your choosing) working harder and faster?
2 Are small compromises in processes and materials sometimes acceptable to get short-term improvements in a measured end-result, including productivity?
3 Can we sometimes improve efficiency and productivity by overlooking some aspects of customer satisfaction?

My answer to each of these questions is "no." If you have read Chapters 1 and 2 and you do not see why I think so, then perhaps my writing is *muda*. In any case, I intend in the rest of this chapter to further illuminate my answer.

Ideas for where to begin looking for *muda* in the NICU

The notion of *muda* implies evaluating the relationship between an activity and its results. Once you explicitly categorize activities according to criteria of systemic value you may never be able to return to former ways of thinking. You may be surprised at what you find when you begin to look for *muda*. Like entropy in a physical system, *muda* seems to occur spontaneously in organizations and processes. Its prevalence can be surprisingly high. Here are some examples of where to look for *muda*:

- the process of admitting a patient to the NICU
- the process of feeding an infant in the NICU

- stocking of instruments, independently of usage rates, on the trays used for catheterizing the umbilicus and inserting a chest tube
- the processes leading from a stat chest x ray request to the developed film in the provider's hand
- the circumstances surrounding unintentional extubation of an infant
- entering the same measurement values in multiple records – data redundancy
- diagnostic testing (the subject of the next chapter).

  - We may discover that some long-accepted diagnostic approaches do not sufficiently improve our level of uncertainty to justify clinical action.

Ideas for reducing *muda*

We may improve efficacy, efficiency, and productivity – and related to all these, customer satisfaction – by one fundamental approach. That way is to reduce or eliminate *muda* from our work. Just as the Inuits have a varied and locally useful assortment of subcategories of "snow", quality improvement and process engineering workers subcategorize waste of resources or activity in operationally useful ways.

Langley *et al* require 66 pages to merely enumerate their concepts for improving a work process![2] Their potentially overwhelming list of ideas is categorized along these lines:

- eliminating waste (some of the subcategories below are closer to the notion of *muda*)
- improving the flow of work
- reducing inventory to reflect true needs
- modifying the work environment
- improving the relationships with the customers and with the suppliers
- using time well
- designing processes to prevent mistakes rather than to correct them
- recognizing the core activities of the work.

Although categorizing may facilitate thinking, for our present purpose the point is to develop sensitivity and skill in identifying and appropriately acting on *muda*. Here are some hospital-based examples inspired by material from Dr Paul B Batalden's course (at the Dartmouth Medical School, Center for the Evaluative Clinical Sciences) on Continual Improvement in Health Care.

We consume resources without adding value when we:

- collect the same patient information more than once
- enter the same information in several places in the medical record and NICU charts
- limit our outcomes research to collecting data about the end-results of our care. This amounts to trying to get a good end-result by inspecting it. (We address this in the chapter on variation. Briefly, outcomes management – inspecting the end result and trying to change subsequent outcomes on the basis of that information – is conceptually insufficient. We can improve end-results by using knowledge of factors that are *upstream* in the causal sequence.)

We consume resources without adding value when we make mistakes we must then redo:

- pharmacy sends the wrong IV bag to the NICU
- blood sample for a drug level obtained at the wrong time
- patient report is filed in the wrong chart
- an unbelievable value for a diagnostic test (for example, total serum calcium level of 0·9 mg/dl).

We consume resources without adding value when we deal with services or supplies we don't need:

- unused hospital beds
- unread professional journals
- maintaining a supply of medications or infant formula without regard to historical pattern of use, resulting in stock that hasn't added value but has reached expiration date.

We consume resources without adding value when we allow unnecessary steps in our work:

- mandatory consults when the evidence does not support such policy
- trip to radiology department for daily review of films when no radiographs were taken since the last review
- specifically notifying a physician of information which clearly will not alter thinking or action.

We consume resources without adding value when we ignore upstream bottlenecks causing delays:

- "7:30 c-section" occurs at 9:00 am because anesthesia is tied up in OR with emergency case
- portable x ray delayed because patient not yet entered in hospital database by admissions office
- delayed meeting time because a participant arrives late.

We consume resources without adding value when we give the customer what they do not need:

- social worker focuses on highest priority problem by her assessment rather than the problem of highest priority to the parent
- stat x ray report provided 24 hours after procedure, although the clinical decision was made five minutes after the x ray was performed
- discharge appointments in conflict with other parent obligations.

I offer so many examples of *muda* because it is highly prevalent and pervasive. You may be skeptical that this generalization applies to your own NICU. I invite you to select any process in your unit, keeping the customer in mind, and analyze it from the point of input through the process steps to completion. You will probably discover *muda*. One respected authority on quality improvement suggests that 95 per cent of all work is waste, while acknowledging that most people would guess the inverse, 5 per cent.[3] We often only see what we look for, so when we look for ideas to improve our work, we must include *muda* in our gaze.

"Drilling down" to reduce *muda*

As you study the process maps you create and plan your improvements, consider these generic change ideas for the processes making up the NICU.[4]

1 Modify the input (for example, work with the perinatologists, take a more active role in choosing supplies, take a more active part in community outreach programs).
2 Combine separate steps (perhaps involving several people) to improve the work flow.
3 Smooth out handoffs between steps (for example, reduce variation among physicians when signing out to each other – use a categorical information checklist).
4 Eliminate a step of questionable added value.
5 Reorder a sequence of steps.
6 Replace a step with a better value alternative.
7 Redesign the process to reflect knowledge of the end-result.
8 Redesign the process to reflect knowledge of the customer.

References

1 Scholtes PR. *The leader's handbook*. New York: McGraw-Hill, 1998.
2 Langley GJ, Nolan KM, Nolan TW, *et al*. *The improvement guide*. San Francisco: Jossey-Bass, 1996.
3 Roberts HV. *A primer on personal quality*. Chicago: Graduate School of Business, University of Chicago, 1995.
4 Batalden PB, Nelson EC. Clinical Improvement Workshop, Hanover, New Hampshire, April 1–3, 1998.

5: Diagnostic testing and *muda*

Let's consider *muda* associated with obtaining information about our patients: consuming resources for diagnostic testing that does not add value to the care. Our scope is limited, with a primary intent to stimulate further interest. We will examine two related areas of medical decision making, test characteristics and Bayesian analysis. If you wish to continue beyond the material we discuss in this chapter, Sox *et al* is a good reference.[1]

Diagnostic tests consume resources and influence subsequent decisions and actions – which again consume resources. Sometimes a clinician's diagnostic testing choices reflect careful reasoning and quantitative analysis, as I shall try to illustrate in this chapter. However, a neonatologist has few tables of NICU-specific test characteristics, needed for such analysis, to refer to. This suggests that at least sometimes, we make uninformed testing decisions. We thus have reason to question the value of the resulting information.

A Bayesian search for *muda* in diagnostic testing

To illustrate some general considerations for evaluating the usefulness of a diagnostic test, let's consider the value of the information provided by the leukocyte esterase test component of a urinalysis. The test characteristics are presented in Table 5.1.[1]

These data are not NICU-specific but they suffice for illustration. Indeed, this chapter will highlight the need to collect this kind of data in the NICU. Pareto charting (see Chapter 7) helps identify the more frequently done tests or the tests that are most expensive – two of the categories we probably want to understand better.

Now, using only the information provided in Table 5.1, please estimate the probability that a patient with a positive result on the leukocyte esterase assay actually has pyuria:

Table 5.1 Leukocyte esterase test component of a urinalysis		
	True-positive rate	**False-positive rate**
Leukocyte esterase assay for pyuria	0·88	0·04

(a) 1
(b) 0·88
(c) approximately 0·5
(d) can't say.

We need more information than appears in the table, so the answer is "d," we can't say.

We undertake diagnostic testing because we wish to improve our level of uncertainty about a patient. Essentially, we hope that the additional information provided by the diagnostic test will support a useful revision of our prior probability estimate of the suspected condition. Therefore, before we undertake diagnostic testing we want to estimate the (prior) probability of the suspected condition. In our example, we require an estimate of the probability of urinary tract infection (UTI) for a newborn (for simplicity, I shall equate UTI with pyuria). The upper limit of the range of incidence of UTI in newborns is about 3%.[2]

Using this additional information, we may now compute the effect of the test result on our uncertainty about the patient's condition (presence of UTI). We do this by applying Bayes' theorem to what we know. A clinically useful way to express Bayes' theorem is in terms of true positive rate (TPR) and false positive rate (FPR), where each of these is defined as follows:

$$\text{True positive rate} = \frac{\text{no. patients with the disease who test positive}}{\text{no. patients with the disease}}$$

$$\text{False positive rate} = \frac{\text{no. patients without the disease who test positive}}{\text{no. patients without the disease}}$$

In general, when we consider the discriminatory power of a test, we are characterizing how well a test can identify a condition, using for comparison the results of a "gold-standard" procedure that operationally defines the true condition of the patient. The *study population*, the patients in whom the test is evaluated, is not the same as the *clinically relevant population*, the patients we typically perform the test upon. Often, the study population is biased (contains systematic error).

- The "gold-standard" may be applied to only the sickest and the healthiest subgroups of the population at risk for the disease.
- The "gold-standard" may be selectively applied to those patients testing positive on the test under evaluation.

As a result:

- The TPR tends to be lower in the clinically relevant population than in the study population.
- Unless the study population was comprised of healthy volunteers, the FPR tends to be lower in the clinically relevant population.

Thus we may reasonably make some (subjective) adjustment in the values we use to compute *posterior probabilities* (the new probability of disease after obtaining the test result).

With the disclaimers made, let's now look at Bayes' formula:

$$\text{Probability of disease if test result is positive} = \frac{\text{probability of disease} \times \text{TPR}}{\{\text{probability of disease} \times \text{TPR}\} + \{(1 - \text{probability of disease}) \times \text{FPR}\}}$$

We now insert the values for the leukocyte esterase test:

$$\text{Probability of UTI if leukocyte esterase test is positive} = \frac{(0.03) \times (0.88)}{\{(0.03) \times (0.88)\} + \{(1 - 0.03) \times 0.04\}}$$
$$= 0.4$$

Or, when we receive a positive leukocyte esterase test report, four times out of ten the patient will actually have a UTI.

Table 5.2   General possibilities for test performance

Diagnostic test result being evaluated	Gold-standard test results		Row totals
	Positive for disease	Negative for disease	
Positive	TP	FP	TP + FP
Negative	FN	TN	FN + TN
Column totals	TP + FN	FP + TN	

Maybe this way is more intuitive

You might find the results of Bayesian probability revision more intuitive if I formulate the reasoning another way. First, let's identify the general possibilities for test performance, as in Table 5.2.

The TPR (defined in the last section) is also known as the *sensitivity* of a test. Using the formulation of this table, we may define TPR as:

$$\frac{TP}{TP + FN}$$

The true negative rate (TNR) is defined as:

$$\frac{TN}{TN + FP}$$

TNR is also known as the *specificity* of a test.

Now let's use the data for the leukocyte esterase test (see Table 5.3). Let's assume our population is 1000 infants. We use a UTI incidence rate of 3% to compute the column totals (see Table 5.4). (The choice of incidence or prevalence rate properly depends on the purpose of the study. We will not discuss this epidemiology issue here.)

We know the TPR is 0·88. Of the 30 infants with UTI having either a positive leukocyte esterase assay or a negative one, 88% will have a positive test result. We compute the number of false negatives by subtracting the number of TP from the total number with UTI (see Table 5.5).

Table 5.3   The leukocyte esterase test; step 1

Leukocyte esterase assay	Gold-standard test results		Row totals
	UTI present	No UTI	
Positive	TP	FP	TP + FP
Negative	FN	TN	FN + TN
Column totals	TP + FN	FP + TN	

Table 5.4   The leukocyte esterase test; step 2

Leukocyte esterase assay	Gold-standard test results		Row totals
	UTI present	No UTI	
Positive	TP	FP	TP + FP
Negative	FN	TN	FN + TN
Column totals	30	970	1000

Table 5.5   The leukocyte esterase test; step 3

Leukocyte esterase assay	Gold-standard test results		Row totals
	UTI present	No UTI	
Positive	26·4	FP	TP + FP
Negative	3·6	TN	FN + TN
Column totals	30	970	

Next, we compute the numbers in the column for no UTI by using the FPR. Of the 970 infants without UTI, 4% will have a positive leukocyte esterase assay (FPR is 0·04). Therefore, 96% of infants without a UTI will have a negative test result (see Table 5.6)

The probability of a UTI if an infant has a positive leukocyte esterase test equals:

$$\frac{\text{no. infants with a positive test that have a UTI by gold standard}}{\text{no. infants with a positive test}}$$

$$= \frac{26\cdot4}{65\cdot2}$$

$$= 0\cdot4$$

Table 5.6 The leukocyte esterase test; step 4			
Leukocyte esterase assay	Gold-standard test results		Row totals
	UTI present	No UTI	
Positive	26·4	38·8	65·2
Negative	3·6	931·2	934·8
Column totals	30	970	1000

This is the same result we obtained earlier. This so-called 2 × 2 table approach makes the subcategories of infants explicit.

Fine, the probability of a UTI in an infant with a positive leukocyte esterase test is 40%, not a more impressive 80%, 90%, or higher. "Even so," you might say, "if there is a 40% chance that my patient has a UTI, that's a pretty good basis for action, so what is different for having gone to the trouble of making the computation we've just labored over?"

The difference that emerges for doing the computation is a function of the disease we are considering. The 3% incidence rate that I used seems rather high for my own experience. What if UTI occurs in only 0·5% of infants? Or, what if we confine ourselves to just the term well-newborn population, and say for the sake of discussion that UTI occurs in 0·3% of these infants. What then happens to the post-test probability?

Let's go back to the Bayes' equation and substitute 0·003 for 0·03. Our new answer is 0·06, or only a 6% probability of a UTI. Here is the take-away message of this (perhaps tedious, but) important computational exercise: *as isolated data, test results cannot be interpreted; independent of other relevant information, test results yield an incomplete picture of a patient's disease status.*

To evaluate the results of a diagnostic test we need specific disease knowledge

The effect of a test result on our estimate of the likelihood of disease depends on the *pretest probability that the patient has the disease!* The lower the probability of disease before a test is performed, the lower will be the computed probability of disease following a positive test result. Exploring these Bayesian insights by recalculating the given example with several different values leads to some important generalizations.[1]

- When pretest disease probability is high, most tests will not substantially help you rule out disease.
- When pretest probability is low (that is, an uncommon occurrence is being considered), most tests will not substantially help you rule in disease.

My point is that Bayesian thinking can provide a framework for some of our improvement efforts. For example, a unit might collect data to describe particular diagnostic test characteristics for the local population and they might also establish the relevant local incidence and prevalence rates. The staff then can thoughtfully work with questions about *muda* associated with using tests so characterized. Since no one benefits from unnecessary testing, this is a way to congruently cut costs and improve care.

Overtreating: a plea for locally determined test characteristics

You say you'd rather err on the conservative side and overtreat if it means not missing a septic infant? At least implicitly, you always establish a threshold value below which you do not consider treatment. But do you think you should be able to explicitly answer the following questions?

- What constitutes an acceptable case identification rate?
- What is the right rate of overtreatment?

Do you believe that surgeons should operate on all cases of possible appendicitis? Or do you accept, and expect, *some* normal appendices on pathological examination, but become concerned when *too many* normals (whatever that number may be) appear during pathology case review. In the context of an outcomes research primer, I do not intend to resolve this issue here, but I do want to stimulate your thoughts on the subject. If you are interested in more detail on this subject, I refer you to Sox *et al.*[1] For our context, I shall continue by framing the issue more specifically for neonatal care providers.

Some workers recently attempted to conduct a meta-analysis of studies that evaluated the accuracy of white blood cell counts (WBC) with differentials and C-reactive protein (CRP) for diagnosing sepsis in the neonate.[3] Because of the consequences of delay in identifying or in actually not identifying a case of sepsis, we tend to treat at a low diagnostic threshold, and thus we probably overtreat many patients. The cited review quotes a 12% rate of positive blood cultures among infants evaluated for possible infection – are only 12% of the appendices removed at your hospital diseased? The authors could not actually perform a meta-analysis because of statistical heterogeneity – they found too much variation among the studies reviewed to allow them to pool the data from each report.

When we identify heterogeneity it means that we cannot assume the individual samples (study results) came from the same population. So, what are the implications for generalizing the results of any of the individual reports that were reviewed for the meta-analysis to your own patient population? The simple answer: You can't do it. Thus, we see the basis and need to evaluate diagnostic tests on a local level.

We can only speculate about how much of our present approach to diagnostic testing represents *muda*.

The receiver operating characteristic (ROC) curve: diagnostic tests and categorical discrimination

Sometimes we have a choice of diagnostic tests when we are trying to reduce our uncertainty about a patient's condition. To minimize *muda* we want to know which test best discriminates those with disease from non-diseased subjects. The receiver operating characteristic (ROC) curve graphically describes the discriminating ability of a test.

Every test entails a trade-off between true positive rate and false positive rate. In the real world, the curves describing the distribution of test results among diseased and non-diseased subjects tend to have some overlap. This means that if we set the threshold value that defines disease at a point where all

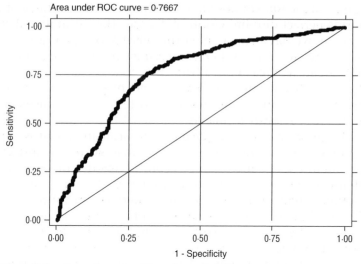

Area under ROC curve = 0·7667

Figure 5.1   A receiver operating characteristic curve

diseased subjects are included, some non-diseased subjects will also have results in this range. Similarly, if we set the threshold of non-disease at a point where all non-diseased are included, some diseased subjects will also have results in this range.

The ROC curve plots TPR on the vertical axis and FPR on the horizontal axis, thus showing how test performance is affected by the "cut-point", the chosen definition of a test result – the measurement value for which disease lies on one side and non-disease on the other. Unless a test is perfect (probably impossible except perhaps for diagnosing death) a cut-point for abnormality that identifies only patients with disease will result in some number of patients with disease but who yield a "normal" test result. If we want to identify all diseased patients, we must lower our cut-point for abnormality, so we must accept some false positives. Figure 5.1 shows an example of a ROC curve.

The 45° line identifies test performance with no ability to discriminate disease from non-disease. The area above the 45° line describes useful test performance – tests whose performance lies in this region can discriminate diseased individuals from non-diseased. The computed area under the curve is a measure of discriminatory power, where a value of 1 means perfect discrimination of disease. The illustrative ROC curve above has an area under the curve of 0·77, considered a good value for a test. When comparing two tests, the test with the greatest area under the ROC curve is the better discriminator. Before employing a new diagnostic test, verify that the ROC curve indicates the new test is an improvement on those previously available.

The cut-point value supplied by a clinical laboratory usually is not an absolute determination. We may want to adjust the threshold for our responding according to the consequences of missing disease or treating normalcy. A more informed method than using statistical dispersion measures, and described in detail in Sox *et al*, accounts for pretest probability and an assessment of costs and benefits to the patient.[1] Instead of a cut-point criterion like two standard deviations from the mean, this approach defines abnormality as that test result that would trigger action, such as treatment, after taking into account the ROC curve, the cost of acting on false positives, and the benefits of acting on true positives.

Recapping

- To accurately estimate the likelihood of disease in a patient by using the results of a diagnostic test, you need knowledge of the test characteristics and of the disease frequency in the population the patient comes from.
- Verify that you have chosen the test with the greatest discriminating power among the testing options.

References

1 Sox HCJ, Blatt MA, Higgins MC, Marton KI. *Medical decision making.* Boston: Butterworth-Heinemann, 1988.
2 Cloherty JP, Stark AR. *Manual of neonatal care.* Philadelphia: Lippincott-Raven, 1998.
3 Da Silva O, Ohlsson A, Kenyon C. Accuracy of leukocyte indices and C-reactive protein for diagnosis of neonatal sepsis: a critical review. *Pediatr Infect Dis J* 1995;14:362–6

6: Needless complexity in our care processes

How needless complexity compounds to undermine process reliability

Suppose you discover that a method or a process used in the NICU is not performing reliably or that the results are unacceptably variable. You might assume that the method or the process is at fault. We will discuss how to quantitatively evaluate process performance in the chapter on variation. For now, let's look at the effect on overall reliability when we add "corrective" steps to what we do, with good intentions but unenlightened about process evaluation.

Adding steps to work makes things more complex. The increased complexity may be of two types.

1 *Linear*: added steps of this type can only fit into the whole in one way. The difference in complexity between a 500-piece jigsaw puzzle and a 1000-piece jigsaw puzzle is one of linear complexity.
2 *Exponential or combinatorial*: added steps of this type can relate to several, or even all, parts of the whole. The possibilities for interaction grow exponentially or combinatorially. Systems growing in this way may become practically unknowable.

For any particular level of reliability for each component, added complexity erodes process or system reliability and quality. Suppose we have a process comprised of a number of basic components or steps, each of which is 99% reliable – that is, it functions as it should 99 times out of 100. If the process has 10 steps, it will perform as expected 9 times in 10 trials. What happens to reliability if the process has 100 steps? Things will go as expected only 4 times in 10. Now, what can we expect from a process with 1000 steps? This number is doubtless far smaller than the total number of process steps comprising the routine function of a busy NICU. Well, when each step is 99% reliable, overall, things will go as expected only *4 times in 100 000!* (That is not a misprint: 4 times in 100 000 is correct.)

Does this quantitation of the effect of increasing complexity surprise you? I offer a mathematical explanation for any skeptics or for those especially interested. The problem represents a straightforward application of the binomial probability distribution. This function describes the frequency distribution of nominal events – events that can occur in one of two states, such as "function properly" or "not function properly." To compute the probability of *k* successes given *N* trials we use the formula:[1]

$$\binom{N}{K} (P)^K (1 - P)^{N-K}$$

Where:

$$\binom{N}{K} = \frac{N!}{K!(N - K)!}$$

$$! = \text{"factorial", for example,}$$
$$3! = (3) \times (2) \times (1)$$
$$= 6$$

And P = probability of occurrence of proper functioning for each component.

So, to compute the probability for a system with individual component P = 0·99 of properly functioning all the time (K = 1000) with 1000 components (N = 1000) we have (reducing expressions):

$$(1) \times (0{\cdot}99)^{1000} (0{\cdot}01)^0 = 0{\cdot}000043171$$

Or, things will go correctly approximately 4 times in 100 000.

I have a hunch that the ideas of combinatorial complexity and reliability as a function of a binomial probability distribution may underlie the notion of *kaizen,* a particular way of improving things that appears in a later chapter. *Kaizen* is the Japanese term describing the steady improvement in system performance resulting from the continual quality improvement methods we discuss in this book. It is a steady improvement that, with each increment, is barely perceptible, but cumulatively becomes quite significant.

Reference

1 Pagano M, Gauvreau K. *Principles of biostatistics.* Belmont, CA: Duxbury Press, 1993.

7: More tools for "drilling down"

Reiterative tests of change: the PDCA cycle

The nature of pediatricians' work gives them a particularly deep appreciation of play. They know that playing is a way of "trying out ideas" in a relatively controlled setting. It is an important way for children to make sense of, and take on a more active role in their world. Properly arranged, it can also be an important way for adults to do the same – to seriously play with a system with the aim of learning about it and achieving a significant degree of mastery of it.

The complex causal webs, the non-linear interdependencies that we've discussed, can define a deterministic but unpredictable system. We can still learn about it however, predictable or not, mold it to be more like what we want, and get it to produce end-results closer to our aims. We poke here and prod there – not doing too many things at once – and then we stand back and observe what happens. Wheatley and Kellner-Rogers speak of "sending pulses into the system to see what it notices."[1]

So let's discuss a systematic way of sending pulses into the system to see what it notices, a way that informs us about the system and leads to improved end-results. This improvement model is called the PDCA cycle – Plan, Do, Check, and Act. (Sometimes the word "Study" replaces "Check", the PDSA cycle – the same model either way.) This model appears commonly in healthcare improvement literature. It works well in a variety of settings but you will also see other models employed.[2]

All theories are wrong, but some are useful.

George Box

All theories are right, in some world.

W Edwards Deming

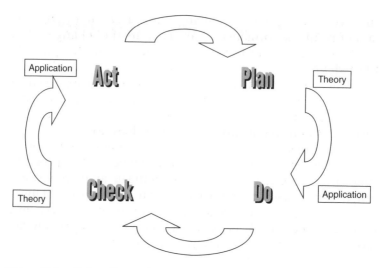

Figure 7.1 Reiterative cycle between theory and application

We can never absolutely prove an inductive theory. At best, we demonstrate successful application until we encounter a contradiction. Here is a theory: "The proper inspiratory time for mechanically ventilating an infant with a pulmonary time constant of x, is y." We must collect appropriate data to substantiate it, to "prove" it, and the proof stands until data appear to refute it.

We do not learn solely from theory or solely from action. We learn from interaction of the two. We start with a hypothesis derived from system knowledge and we collect appropriate data to establish some "proof". We do this in a reiterative cycle (see Figure 7.1).

We cycle between theory and application. *This is how we test a change to a system,* such as a change idea stemming from concepts in the chapters on *muda, and how we learn from the results of the test.* Ever mindful of operational definitions, we specify how we determine that a change represents an improvement – some changes may turn out to represent quite the opposite result. Mindful of the system aim, we also state explicitly what we wish to achieve by this change.

In this way, we keep "rolling along." We plan a change after understanding what we can about the process we want to improve – mapping it, looking for *muda*, analyzing the variation in performance. We try out the change idea, checking the effect of the change by measuring thoughtfully selected upstream and downstream outcome variables and applying pre-determined decision rules for evaluating the data we collect. Then we act on our new knowledge – making the change part of a new routine if it improves the outcomes, rejecting it and trying another idea if it does not.

Each complete turn of the PDCA cycle builds knowledge of our system, so perhaps it is more accurate to think of the trajectory as a spiral. Others speak of rolling up an improvement ramp.[3] Some aspect of the NICU system is always changing – inputs, processes, the operating environment, budgets, etc. Therefore, the PDCA cycle must always be kept moving, becoming a regular part of the daily work in the NICU.

Cause and effect diagram: formulating a "differential diagnosis" for an outcome

Process mapping and cause and effect diagramming each inform us about a process, but they provide different information. Process mapping helps us understand *how* a process unfolds, what happens when, and by whom. Creating a cause and effect diagram helps us understand *why* the process produces a particular effect.

More specifically, the aim of cause and effect diagramming is to identify an upstream root cause for a downstream manifestation. Keeping this in mind, we therefore try to distinguish the history of a problem from the content of the problem. Also, the presenting problem may not be the problem to solve. Let's take an example from clinical practice: an infant is fussy for several days before manifesting seizures. We investigate the underlying etiology and do not treat based only on the manifestation of the problem (the symptom) and preceding historical events. We know, for instance, that treating an infant with seizures caused by pyridoxine deficiency differs from treating an infant with seizures caused by bacterial meningitis.

So a cause and effect diagram – also known as a fishbone diagram (for obvious reasons when you look at Figure 7.2) or an Ishikawa diagram (named after a leading Japanese figure in

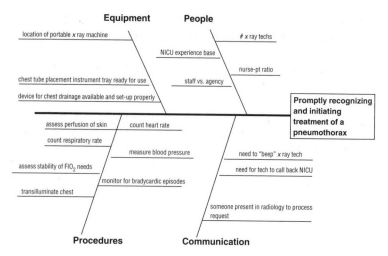

Figure 7.2   Cause and effect diagram showing possible factors relating to promptly recognizing and treating pneumothorax

system improvement work) – is a diagrammatic differential diagnosis of an outcome. Note that an outcome need not be an end-result.

Physicians are accustomed to formulating a differential diagnosis (of a clinical outcome for a particular patient) occasionally in collaboration with other physicians but often as an independent activity. A systems approach calls for integrating as many relevant perspectives as are available. Include many people involved with the process. Since we often only see what we look for, multiple knowledgeable participants produce a higher dimensional model – one that includes more information about the current reality than would result from fewer perspectives.

Figure 7.2 presents an example of a cause and effect diagram created to help understand how to improve the way pneumothorax is identified and treated in a hypothetical NICU. No doubt you will be able to think of additional "bones" and factors to consider.

Here are some tips for making a cause and effect diagram:[4,5]

1   Assemble those who know the process that is associated with the effect (outcome) under study.

2 Agree on explicit language describing the effect.

3 Place the description of the effect (outcome) on the right side of the charting area.

4 Invite each person to brainstorm possible causes. Use Post-it notes for each suggestion so ideas may be easily rearranged.

5 Have a working surface with plenty of room for expanding the diagram, and have it in easy view of all.

6 Create the major "bones" coming off of the central "vertebral column" to correspond with general categories for causes, and label these "bones." Consider categories such as:

- people
- equipment
- materials
- environment
- timing
- communication
- policies
- procedures
- measurements.

7 Be flexible about how you categorize causes. Make the diagram categories fit the problem.

8 The aim at this stage is to develop as wide an array of possibilities as you can.

9 Attach each Post-it Note naming a possible cause to the appropriate category bone. Some further branching into subcategories may be logically appropriate. (This is not shown on the illustration.)

10 Remember that the aim of the exercise is to uncover *root causes* for an effect. You want to *"drill down"* into a problem.

11 Ask "Why does this happen?" for a suggested cause and/or "What could happen because of this cause?" This may reveal new possibilities. Also, doing this on one causal point, for several iterations, may be productive – you are looking for the *root* cause, and that may lie several branch points upstream. The Japanese approach cause and effect problems by asking "Why?" five times. I think of this approach as exponentiating a question (here, to the fifth power).

12 Include or eliminate possibilities by using some evidence-based assessment of reality and not, for example, by "expert" (but unsubstantiated) authority.

- Use explicit, mutually agreed-upon decision rules.
- Watch for causes appearing in more than one place.
- Gather data on the relative frequency of the possibilities, creating a Pareto chart, which we discuss in the next section.

13 Don't hide the diagram in a closet after creating it. Keep it out in view, so that people can add to it as they get more experience.

14 Keep an open mind. What at first looks promising may turn out not to be. Consider running tests of alternative hypotheses.

Pareto charting

A Pareto diagram is a frequency distribution histogram displaying the relative importance of a number of things under study. The diagram facilitates applying the Pareto Principle, also known as the 80/20 rule. Simply stated: 80% of the trouble typically comes from 20% of the problems.[2] Even when things appear to be overwhelmingly chaotic, don't underestimate the potential of a careful, systematic approach to problem solving. Once we discover the usual sources of a problem, concentrating the improvement effort on a few well chosen areas can have great positive effect. Arranging the items in descending order on the x-axis, we create an easy-to-read chart that shows rank order of importance. This tool is helpful at many stages of improvement work.

- Rank ordering of system problems.
- Rank ordering of causes of a selected problem (effect, outcome).
- Displaying progress – a Pareto diagram to show the situation before and after instituting a change.

Since processes unfold over time, we may ask what is the proper time period for the study. "Collect data over enough time to represent the situation," sounds good but we must operationally define our terms – and these will vary with the context. Data from times other than our collection period may not be similar. The highest-ranked problem may be severe but occur infrequently and coincidentally during our data collection period, or it may be a lower-grade problem and occur chronically. So you can see why collecting data independent of process knowledge carries great risk of error.

Consider for example, a Pareto diagram of causes of medication errors in the NICU of a teaching hospital. Rankings and causes for study periods July–September, April–June, and July–June might all differ. We can learn about the time pattern of occurrence by plotting the data for each x-axis item as a run chart – the next tool in this section. When we forget this potential for variation in the time pattern of occurrence we risk sending our problem-solving efforts off in the wrong direction. *We want to verify that the identified rankings and causes are typical.*

Here is a sequence of steps for creating a Pareto diagram that includes an optional cumulative percentage line plot by using Microsoft Excel:

1 Enter the categories and their respective counts.
2 Sort descending.
3 Compute total occurrences.
4 Compute the cumulative occurrences.
5 Compute cumulative percentages.

   • Format the column to show percentage values; verify that the total is 100%.

6 Select the columns for plotting.
7 Click on the chart wizard button.
8 Follow the prompts, selecting the bar and line chart with a right (# occurrences for each category) and a left (cumulative %) axis.

Table 7.1 illustrates what these steps produce, using fictional data. Figure 7.3 is the chart produced from these data.

Did you notice that the data do not conform to the Pareto Principle (80% of the trouble comes from 20% of the problems)? The rule often holds up for statistically stable systems (that is, predictable, and with no identifiable external influences – see Chapter 10 on understanding variation). System data may, however, describe unpredictable, poorly characterized systems.

Table 7.1   Characteristics of patients with nosocomial infection

Characteristic	Occurrences	Cumulative occurrences	Cumulative %
Steroids	63	63	23%
<1000 g	52	115	43%
Intubated	42	157	58%
1 central line	37	194	72%
TPN	34	228	85%
Indomethacin	17	245	91%
Invasive procedures	17	262	97%
2 central lines	7	269	100%
Total occurrence	269		

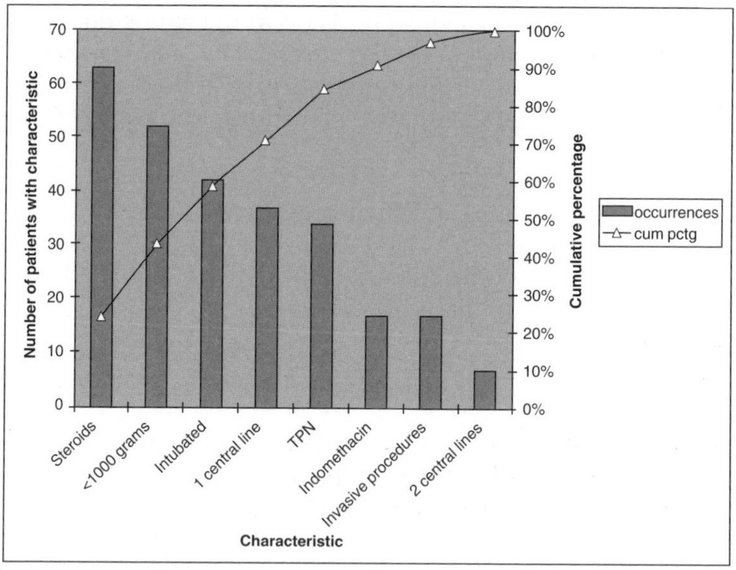

Figure 7.3   Pareto chart of characteristics of patients at time of nosocomial infection

Also, raw data are often "dirty" – the set contains erroneous values. Sometimes, and possibly the case in this example, we may start off by inadvertently considering more than one system or process simultaneously, that is, neglecting to stratify the data. Thus, perhaps considering the data separately for each birth weight category (for example, 500–750 grams, 751–1000 grams, etc.) might be more informative. Or perhaps our bins (the

Table 7.2 List of temperature measurements

Time order sequence	Measurement value	Time order sequence	Measurement value
1	37·5	26	37·46
2	37·51	27	37·42
3	37·505	28	37·44
4	37·49	29	37·43
5	37·5	30	37·46
6	37·43	31	37·42
7	37·42	32	37·43
8	37·45	33	37·42
9	37·47	34	37·45
10	37·49	35	37·49
11	37·46	36	37·5
12	37·5	37	37·51
13	37·52	38	37·52
14	37·525	39	37·54
15	37·51	40	37·51
16	37·52	41	37·49
17	37·5	42	37·5
18	37·49	43	37·495
19	37·54	44	37·51
20	37·51	45	37·5
21	37·52	46	37·52
22	37·46	47	37·5
23	37·42	48	37·48
24	37·43	49	37·495
25	37·45	50	37·49

categories defined by the x-axis label of the bars) are not appropriately set up. Perhaps "invasive procedures" should include the separate bins for central lines.

The run chart: preserving the time dimension

The time dimension is an important aspect of understanding what is happening in a system. But often we collect data over weeks, months, or even longer periods and then summarize it by computing the central tendency and a measure of dispersion (the mean and standard deviation), thus describing the distribution of the values. We often do this because summarizing raw data helps us manage a large data set. Table 7.2 gives a list of temperature measurements (for the present

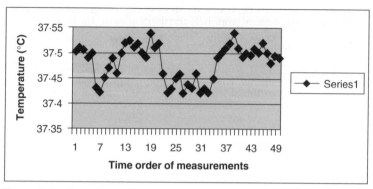

Figure 7.4   Run chart of temperature measurements

purpose, set aside the issue that the differences are clinically insignificant).

What can you say about the information contained in the raw data? I tried to make it easy for you by listing the data in columns. The run chart shown in Figure 7.4 contains the same information. Does this display facilitate your understanding of the data? Notice too, with this format no information is lost (that is, we retain the time ordering of the data).

A run chart is a running record of process measurements *over time*. Interesting and important changes occurring in the course of events are evident. No data are compressed and no dimensions are eliminated. We aren't actually doing anything to the data. We are just usefully displaying it. Displaying data on a run chart facilitates identifying trends, shifts, and cycles. If we plot "before and after" data, we can make quick eyeball assessments. But how do we decide on threshold criteria for identifying those trends, shifts, and cycles? The techniques of statistical process control (SPC) for understanding variation in measurements help us answer that question. We turn to this subject soon.

References

1   Wheatley MJ, Kellner-Rogers M. *A simpler way*. San Francisco, CA: Berrett-Koehler, 1996.
2   Scholtes PR. *The leader's handbook*. New York: McGraw-Hill, 1998.

3   Nelson EC, Batalden PB, Plume SK, Mohr JJ. Improving health care. Part 2: A clinical improvement worksheet and user's manual. *The Joint Commission Journal on Quality Improvement* 1996;**22**:531–48.
4   Brassard M, Ritter D. *The memory jogger II*. Methuen, MA: GOAL/QPC, 1994.
5   Jordan JA, Jordan LM, Ranney GB. *Methods for continual improvement with applications to health care*. Limited distribution; copy provided by The Center for the Evaluative Clinical Sciences at Dartmouth Medical School, 1997.

Part 2:
Data

When you can measure what you are speaking about, and express it
in numbers, you know something about it.

Lord Kelvin

8: Measuring outcomes: What? How?

Toward an operational definition of "outcomes research"

I've been circumspect with the term "outcomes research" – avoiding it, actually – but we are now prepared to explicitly discuss this concept. Why did I delay introducing a term that appears in the subtitle of this book? In the neonatology literature "outcomes research" is often operationally undefined, an inexact term.[1] And I fear that the benefits of conducting outcomes research may diminish in proportion to the participant's conceptual ambiguity surrounding the activity. I hope that by first understanding our work as a system we may arrive at a more definite and useful concept of outcomes research.

Published outcomes research commonly reports on only a few selected end-results of the work we do in NICUs – the measured outcomes are often mortality and a few types of morbidity rates.[1]

- This may dispose toward a conceptual and operational focus solely on end-results. Of course, we care a great deal about the way things turn out. But end-results do not inform us about what may have gone wrong or how we may improve those results.
- Because a process error does not invariably lead to a measurable effect on the end-result, we may miss important information by only observing what is happening "downstream."

Suppose we review last year's mortality rates, along with incidence rates for bronchopulmonary dysplasia (BPD), necrotizing enterocolitis (NEC), and pneumothorax (PTX). Perhaps we compare them with values for similar measures from a colleague's unit. If we think our numbers are "good," what do we do next? How do we respond if we think our numbers are not "good"? These determinations are informed by upstream process knowledge. Making comparative assessments – before and after a change, their NICU and ours – calls for making measurements. So we now consider how to choose the variables to measure and how to measure the variables we choose.

Why, fundamentally, do we measure whatever it is we measure in the NICU? We want to know how well our patients are doing. (Operational definitions are often embedded in standards of care, but sometimes the definitions must be locally established.) And why do we want to know how our patients are doing? We may have several reasons including wanting to ascertain that the results of our work are at least as good as are the results of our respected colleagues. If our results are not as good, we undoubtedly want to improve upon what we are doing. And what if our results are comparable to, or are better than those of our respected colleagues? Are we confident that our comparisons are appropriate and fair? (Of course, we want to ascertain this in all cases.) If so, what then? Do we leave things as they are? Would we accept today outcome measures reported from the best units of 20 years ago? Clearly, the answer is "no." We seek to learn about our work so that our results continue to improve.

Recall the earlier proposal of "efficacy" as doing the right thing; I also consider this appropriate care. And we've referred to "efficiency" as doing the right thing well; this I consider appropriately provided care. (Again, first we need process-specific operational definitions. These can range from an individual NICU formulation to perhaps a statement by the American Academy of Pediatrics.) Providing appropriate care is necessary but not sufficient for achieving the best possible outcomes. We must appropriately provide the appropriate care. We may say, then, that outcomes research concerns itself with determining that appropriate care is being appropriately provided – that what we do is both effective and efficient.

In this light, we may consider "outcomes research" as research into thoughtfully selected end-results and their associated – often obscure – upstream causal factors. Any of the input, intermediary-process, or end-results measurement variables that we select may be termed an "outcome," because in the measurement context it is a selected end-result. Thus, "systems research" might more accurately describe our activities for understanding and improving the results of our work, but at least we now have greater clarity about the denotation of "outcomes research."

What do we want to measure? Well, what question are we asking?

Let's now add specificity to the question "What should we measure?" In addition to knowing how things turn out, we also ask: "How do we identify measurable leverage points that importantly account for the end-results of our work processes?"

A systems perspective justifies skepticism of preliminary problem assessments. We know that often the presenting problem may not resemble the real problem.[2] We examined this observation closely when we discussed cause and effect diagrams. Similarly, we must distinguish data that are easily available from the data that are truly informative. For example, measuring blood pressure is easier than measuring cardiac output. We often use blood pressure data as a proxy for cardiac output data. This substitution usually does not degrade our process of deduction but sometimes we must directly measure what we actually need to know. When we use a proxy variable for reasoning about causes and effects related to the actual variable of interest we may ultimately arrive at an erroneous conclusion.

Our decisions about what we should measure derive from knowledge of the NICU as a system and the problems that each NICU identifies. We face at least three challenges:

1 We need to know how to identify our problems.
2 We need to know how to choose those upstream steps causally linked with the problem manifestation itself.
3 We need to quantitatively assess the variables associated with items 1 and 2.

The material we thus far have worked through is still not all we need for succeeding with these challenges. We next consider compartmentalizing our work perspective; this can

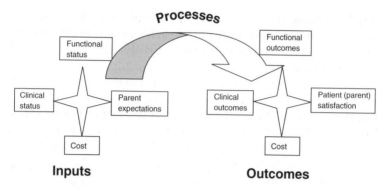

Figure 8.1 A formulation of the clinical value compass, adapted from Nelson EC, *et al*. *The Joint Commission Journal on Quality Improvement* 1996;**22**:243–58.[3]

help guide us toward identifying the "measurable leverage points importantly accounting for the end-results of our work processes."

The clinical value compass and NICU outcomes

To determine whether we are providing appropriate care, we seek an array of measures that resonate with the aims of the system (NICU) we are evaluating. Trying to characterize or evaluate our system by merely one or a very few measures, we deceive ourselves with oversimplification, incompleteness, and superficiality. We seek an array balanced in its focus, manageably small, but informing us about possible causal factors and the end-results of interest. A practical model for such an approach to performance measurement is the clinical value compass.[3] Figure 8.1 shows how the model explicitly compartmentalizes and interrelates key aspects of NICU activity.

This perspective for choosing what to measure encourages explicit systems thinking – understanding what enters the NICU, understanding what happens to change the inputs, and understanding the end-results, that is, how we are doing. Such data can provide a balanced picture of NICU performance; not just informing us about selected clinical outcomes, but also about the resources we consume to achieve our results and the impact of all the activities on those involved. We must carefully take account of the inputs to our NICU. For instance, maternal status and infant status vary with each individual. Some aspects of environment and personnel may not be constant. We must be aware of these things and adjust for them in both our processes and how we interpret outcomes. Risk adjusting is one such accounting method – beyond the scope of this book but necessary when studying data resulting from varying inputs.[4]

For a balanced picture of how things are going in the NICU we also consider clinical outcomes, functional outcomes, patient satisfaction, and the cost of a patient interacting with our system (resource use). Functional status measures that are useful for characterizing infants in the NICU are rudimentary or non-existent – here is fertile ground for research and improvement.[5] Assessing patient (parent) satisfaction involves seeing the NICU the way those we serve see it. To some extent this requires thinking like a baby and thinking like parents. When you do this you may be surprised at how quickly you think of ideas for process improvement. Costs are important outcome measures, not just for payers. Costs vary with the reference frame, but we must consider all costs if we are genuinely concerned about how well we are doing. Resources used are resources no longer available for other purposes.

Table 8.1 illustrates a value compass formulation for a NICU. Each NICU's formulation will, of course, vary somewhat.

Measuring patient satisfaction is listening to the voice of the customer. In my experience, NICUs don't take a very active role in asking parents how things should be run. If your first response to this is: "Of course not," I invite you to think further about the ways that parents can point us toward better ways of doing our work. As objects of our processes, parents see the work of the NICU in ways that involved professionals may not. Parents have implicit and explicit expectations about our work and the results of their infant receiving care in the NICU. If we aim to please parents and their infants, then excluding their valuable feedback from our evaluative approach simply makes it harder for us to achieve our aim.

Table 8.1   A value compass formulation for a NICU

Value compass point	NICU examples
Clinical outcomes	Death Surgical ligation of patent ductus arteriosus Bronchopulmonary dysplasia Necrotizing enterocolitis Grade IV intraventricular hemorrhage
Functional outcomes	Need for home O_2 Difficult infant to feed by mouth Feeding gastrostomy Infant with inconsolable disposition Routine newborn home care
Satisfaction with care	Parental assessment of: • emotional support provided by staff • timely, effective, and compassionate communication • the transition to outpatient care
Cost	Direct out-of-pocket costs to family Costs to third party payer Unreimbursed costs to hospital Hospital charges for week #1 Hospital charges for a week as a stable, "feeder-grower" premature infant Indirect costs including: • parental time lost from work • transportation to NICU • baby-sitter for children at home

Tips for creating variables to measure

- *Work with internal and external benchmarks* (see Chapter 11). Since you may not know what you don't know, be mindful about being trapped by your own experience. (You may have to think about this for a moment.) Ask others not caught up in your own work and perspectives to judge and to verify your decision rules.
- *Ask your customers what they think of your system.*

  - Be careful to stay on track, focus on the "main book of business," the *Gemba*.
  - Use satisfaction surveys; make them event specific and/or process specific – this will provide data that you can act on.

- *Drill down into your processes.* When you've identified a problem area, gather detailed process knowledge. Map the processes. Use cause and effect diagrams for upstream understanding of the problem area, and Pareto charting to prioritize among the possibilities for further investigation and tests of change.
- *Looking for a "smoking gun" hinders your efforts.* Don't be surprised if you have trouble identifying an obvious causal factor, especially if your NICU has a long history. Instead, look for small foci here and there, not necessarily by themselves exciting but believably relevant. The results initially may be small but the gains will compound. Improvement may seem almost invisible for a while, but by persisting in this way, end-results clearly get better. Recall the discussion of the *muda* of needless complexity and of *kaizen.*
- *Be careful about getting distracted by outliers.* These data points usually don't tell you as much about the process as does the bulk of the distribution. Remember that chance alone may put some of the data points in the tails of the distribution.
- *Verify that you can act on the data coming from your chosen measurements.* Instead of waiting months for results, make up some "dummy data." Verify that you have clear ideas about what to do in response to a variety of fictional but possible measurement values.
- *Recognize explicitly whether your measurement choice focuses on the minority of patients or the majority of patients* that go through the NICU, and verify that is the way you want it. For example, from a mortality rate measurement of 2%, an NICU team decided to focus on deaths in the unit. They could have alternatively chosen to focus on the 98% of patients surviving and the correspondingly different relevant measures for this group.
- *Beware of going off in too many directions at once.* There is a profound difference between improvement work and Brownian movement (I thank Dr Gerald T. O'Connor for this observation). Keep to a very few measures aimed at either identifying an area of possible change or identifying that a change represents an improvement.
  - *Frequently remind yourself that data are everywhere.* You can easily produce an overwhelming variety and

amount of data. Remain ever mindful of your purpose in measuring things. You want information to help answer specific, explicitly stated questions about how your NICU is doing.

- *Ask yourself: "What would be different if we knew this thing?"* If your answer is vague, watch out for *muda*.
- *Think about the upstream process variables that contribute to explaining an end-result.* For example, various organizations commonly measure length of stay (LOS) in the hospital. This is an end-result of many process variables and cannot be safely and reasonably managed solely with knowledge of LOS. Safely influencing this measurement may require data about such things as duration of mechanical ventilation, number of days to full enteric feedings, date of initiation of discharge planning, and so on. Further, "drilling down" for each of these factors will likely also yield helpful insights.

  - *Are we collecting data that inform us about why we are getting the rates we see?* Regression models can inform us of the relative explanatory power of a particular variable. These models are briefly introduced in a later section (for extensive discussion, see Iezzoni,[4] Pagano and Gauvreau,[6] and Kleinbaum *et al* [7]).

- *When possible, disaggregate what you measure – stratify the data.* When you combine measurements of subgroups differing among each other (in ways you may not initially appreciate are relevant) you may obscure main effects that you seek to identify. Differences among the subgroups may even cancel each other out when all the measurements are aggregated. Indeed, since the work of the NICU itself is a complex aggregation of implicit and explicit processes and also of inputs, unbundling facilitates understanding.
- *When you think you've identified what you will measure, ask yourself: "If we measure these things, will we understand better what is going on here? How so?"* Again, a vague answer warns of *muda*.

Investigative perspective and outcome interpretation

Be mindful of making implicit value judgments regarding the outcomes you study, for such (unconscious) thinking can distort what you learn from your data. Here's an interesting illustration. We know that some NICU survivors have significant childhood functional difficulties. Parents and others often ask us about the burdens for such affected children as well as for society. Studies of long-term neurological outcomes of NICU patients may describe sequelae and at the same time frame such descriptions of functional status using implicit value judgments.[8] I refer here to views that frame functional neurologic sequelae as burdens, tragedies. This latter approach, and it is a common one, seems to assume only one possible perspective on the measured outcomes – the investigator's (perhaps corresponding to that of society at large).

However, measuring functional outcomes from the perspective of the patient can yield striking insight: NICU survivors with significantly more functional limitations than the control children have essentially the same perceptions about the quality of their life as do the controls![9] These disabled children attach a higher value to their particular health state, than would children characterized as normal. People adapt to their reality. Since there is no absolute, invariant frame of reference, we must not confuse the physician's perspective for example, with the one that may matter most to the affected individual, that is, that same individual's perspective.

Measuring variables: how?

Measurement methods begin with operational definitions. Useful definitions reflect knowledge of the NICU and its aims, its processes, relevant epidemiology, and statistical analysis. (Some NICUs may find statistical and epidemiological consultative assistance helpful during some portions of their improvement efforts.) In general, how we measure a variable should reflect why we are measuring it.

Depending on the reason for collecting the data, therefore, we may use different measurement units for a particular outcome (remember the clinical value compass and the different perspectives from which we may view outcomes for a single patient). For example, suppose we are interested in survival among a particular stratum of infants in our NICU.

We may measure days until expiration or we may measure units of resource use, such as dollars spent per surviving patient.

Answering these questions can facilitate your work on a chosen outcome.

- *Are the system aims and the measurement method congruent?* This is a broader formulation of connecting how we measure a variable with why we measure it.
- *Have you thought carefully about the unit of measurement?* Does the choice of unit reflect the measurement purpose?
- *Have you made the unit of analysis explicit?* For example – an infant, a cohort, a nursing shift.
- *Have you properly chosen the unit of analysis?* Recall the admonition about thoughtlessly aggregating data. A unit of analysis may contain several measurement variables, and you may want to stratify the data set by one or more of these. When the analysis process lumps, rather than stratifies, subgroups that yield different process results, important main effects in the subgroups may be obscured. Just because all collected data are preserved does not assure against information loss.
- *If you stratified the data, does working with the amount of data contained by all the strata seem cumbersome?* As the number of groups in the analysis rises, you may find that comparing group-specific rates becomes tedious and recognizing patterns becomes harder. You can summarize stratified results by either directly or indirectly standardizing the data – essentially, computing weighted averages that preserve group-specific information. The terms "direct" and "indirect" refer to the source of rate information for the weighting. The source is group-specific for the direct method; rate information comes from a standard population for the indirect method. When each stratum is small in number, changes affecting only one or two individual measurements may have a large effect on the corresponding rate. So for small group size, indirect standardization may result in more reliable summary computations.
- *Does the size of the data set limit the extent to which you can stratify?* When you "slice and dice" into small groups, you

will need to identify larger main effects in order to make valid inference.

- *Is the data-collecting frequency consistent with the process we are monitoring?* For example, measuring numbers of unintended extubations each week might be more informative than doing so in three-month intervals.
- *Are rates the quotient of an appropriately chosen numerator and denominator?*[10] We want to be explicit about what we quantitate, for example, events or individuals, population at risk or total population. Also, a time measurement is an essential part of the denominator, for example, annual mortality rate.

Understanding relationships among variables and comparing data from different NICUs (systems)

Readers of this book undoubtedly appreciate the potential for variation among NICUs and among the populations they serve. Have you ever overheard something like the following exchange? "Yes, NICU A has the lowest bronchopulmonary dysplasia incidence rate we know of, but our rate is higher because our patients are sicker." Of course, such a contention requires supporting data and analysis.

To learn from what our colleagues are doing, to make fair comparisons among NICUs, we need to account for the factors that can affect the variables we are judging. We do this by "risk adjusting," typically using statistical regression techniques.[6,7] Regression models describe the contribution a selected (independent, or predictor) variable makes to the variation observed in the measured values of the outcome variable under study (dependent, or end-result variable). In practice, adjusting for individual risk is difficult and fraught with problems; methods for standardizing data can vary among organizations and regions.[4,11,12]

Sometimes associations between an independent variable and an outcome under study may be only apparent, not real. Although we sidestep regression theory and method in this book, recognizing the basic ways we may err in thinking about causal relationships is fundamentally important for outcomes research. The mistakes typically fit one of three categories.[6,7,10]

- *Confounding* – the influence of an independently associated third variable on both an upstream factor and an outcome. Remove the contribution of the confounding variable and the original apparent association disappears.

- To make inferences about the quality of care we risk adjust for input variables such as severity of illness. The variation remaining after risk adjusting can then be attributed to the care processes. However, substandard care can affect severity of illness. Risk adjusting for severity of illness may obscure (confound) the true association between outcome and NICU care unless our measure of illness severity is carefully designed. This is one reason such illness measures as the score for neonatal acute physiology (SNAP) and clinical risk index for babies (CRIB) scores are implemented soon after birth.[11,12]

- *Interacting variables*, or *effect modifiers* – these are variables that change the effect of an upstream factor on an outcome; for example, gender is an effect modifier for the relationship between respiratory distress syndrome (RDS) and survival.

- *Aggregating groups without regard to the populations from which they are sampled*; data analysis must include thoughtful stratification, informed by context knowledge.

Earlier, I alluded to problems associated with trying to "manage" length of stay (LOS), noting specifically that end-results often do not inform us about how to change those end-results. I can now mention a more meaningful way to work with LOS. We can predict median LOS from a Cox proportional hazards model, a type of regression technique. Although it calls for substantial understanding of statistical theory and technique, this approach may identify upstream variables with significant explanatory power for the observed variation in LOS; thus informing us how to positively influence this outcome measure.[13]

Working with cause and effect diagrams and Pareto charts can help identify which variables we want to study in regression models. Statistical software packages are now so easy to run that we must not mistake computed output for correct analysis; there is real danger in inappropriately selecting or setting-up a statistical routine. Several sources of statistical software appear in the final chapter. Readers requiring, but without access to, statistical consultative support may find the InStat software package to be accessible and helpful for data set-up and test selection.

Lest I overstate the importance of regression analysis for local improvement work, I wish to make clear your initial outcomes research efforts will probably not require regression techniques. If you are interested in only one system (that is, no comparisons) and the process under study is statistically stable (see Chapter 10 on understanding variation), then risk adjusting is not necessary for making valid inferences from the data.

References

1   McCormick MC. The outcomes of very low birth weight infants: are we asking the right questions? *Pediatrics* 1997;**99**:869–76.
2   Block P. *Flawless consulting*. San Francisco, CA: Pfeiffer & Company, 1981.
3   Nelson EC, Mohr JJ, Batalden PB, Plume SK. Improving health care, Part 1: The clinical value compass. *The Joint Commission Journal on Quality Improvement* 1996;**22**:243–58.
4   Iezzoni LI, ed. *Risk adjusting for measuring healthcare outcomes*. Chicago, IL: Health Administration Press, 1997.
5   McCormick MC. Quality of care: an overdue agenda. *Pediatrics* 1997;**99**:249–50.
6   Pagano M, Gauvreau K. *Principles of biostatistics*. Belmont, CA: Duxbury Press, 1993.
7   Kleinbaum DG, Kupper LL, Muller KE, Nizam A. *Applied regression analysis and other multivariable methods*. Pacific Grove, CA: Duxbury Press, 1998.
8   Hack M, Taylor HG, Klein N, *et al*. School-age outcomes in children with birth weights under 750 g. *N Engl J Med* 1994;**331**:753–9.
9   Saigal S, Feeny D, Rosenbaum P, *et al*. Self-perceived health status and health-related quality of life of extremely low-birth-weight infants at adolescence. *JAMA* 1996;**276**:453–9.
10 Hennekens CH, Buring JE. *Epidemiology in medicine*. Boston, MA: Little, Brown and Company, 1987.
11 Richardson DK, Gray JE, McCormick MC, *et al*. Score for neonatal acute physiology: a physiologic severity index for neonatal intensive care. *Pediatrics* 1993;**91**:617–23.
12 The International Neonatal Network. The CRIB (clinical risk index for babies) score: a tool for assessing initial neonatal risk and comparing performance of neonatal intensive care units. *Lancet* 1993;**342**:193–8.
13 Schulman J. Prediction of length of hospital stay in neonatal units for very low birth weight infants (letter). *J Perinatol* 1999;**19**:613.

9: Characterizing variation in our measurements

We act on data that continually varies

When examined with enough precision, we find that no production cycle yields *exactly* the same results every time it operates. Reiterative process results *always* vary.[1,2] Yet we make inferences from those results; and from those inferences, we take action. Every time we seek to learn something from a reiterative process we therefore face an extremely important task: *picking out signals from noise.*

Can you think of a single measurement performed in the NICU that returns exactly the same value every time we look? Think about this using an individual clinically stable patient as your unit of analysis. Blood gases vary with each determination. Complete blood count (CBC) results are never the same. Weight changes daily (if it doesn't appear to, we're not using enough significant digits). Inferentially stated, this serial variation occurs with any variable we choose. Despite this "built-in" variation, we somehow can look at an assortment of values and categorize them: normal or abnormal, actionable or not, "needs watching" or "looks OK." How do we do this? Don't consider this question rhetorical – try to answer it. Can you explicitly describe your decision rules for all data that you judge? Shouldn't your answer be yes?(!)

Filtering data: appropriate responses *v* tampering

Paraphrasing Berwick, neonatologists "measure and change, measure and change."[3] How do we know when a measured value *"means something"*?

We want to avoid mistaking noise for a signal and mistaking a signal for noise. This chapter discusses the techniques of control charting. These tools filter data – they separate signal from noise – and they characterize the process-related data – they distinguish predictable from unpredictable processes.

When we respond to a measurement value as if it is a signal when it is actually noise, we take unnecessary action (*muda*). Engineers call this *tampering*. *Tampering increases the variability* in system or process performance.[4,5] In the NICU, for example, we change aspects of therapy in response to a measurement result, then we measure again, and so on. Presumably, every measurement value prompting a response is an instance of a value that "means something." By adjusting therapy when the result really represents only noise, we can actually *decrease* patient stability. *Minimizing overreaction to natural fluctuations is fundamental to improving neonatal care.*

Decision rules for filtering data: what are we assuming?

Our daily, implicit processes of filtering data may rest upon several assumptions.

- We assume that we are dealing with predictable processes, biological or not (we will return to this notion).
- We assume that the cutpoints we apply for categorizing values (for example, non-disease *v* disease) are unambiguous, meaningful, and appropriate for making important decisions about action or inaction.

  - We often assume that these categorical cutpoints, for whatever we are observing as it unfolds over time, reliably distinguish expected from unexpected performance.

Categorical cutpoints supplied by clinical laboratories, for example, may derive from summary statistics of a sample from a population. Let's say 100 or 1000 infants have a serum enzyme assay performed. The lab may describe the assortment (distribution) of values by a measure of the central tendency of the distribution of values, the mean, and by a measure of the dispersion of the values across their entire range, the standard deviation. Characterizing values outside the central 95% of the distribution as abnormal, for example, one time in twenty puts some individuals in this outlier range just by sampling error. Put differently, with such a cutpoint decision rule, we expect, *by chance alone*, to find an abnormal value among a panel of twenty tests. To account for this reality, multiple comparisons among population samples require special statistical adjustments.

Characterizing processes

Measuring a process as it unfolds over time entails recording the time order of the data. When we compute summary statistics such as the mean and standard deviation we destroy this *time dimension* of our data and we may reach erroneous conclusions about performance.

Here are some questions we want to be able to answer about our work processes.

- How do we know that a series of measurements obtained over time reflects a single process and therefore does not require stratification? Some end-results we measure may reflect more than one process unfolding over time. For example, we measure the time needed to feed an infant. This result may be different if the unit of analysis is the NICU or the unit of analysis is the nursing shift. Perhaps the night shift has a lower measured value because their process is not the same as the day shift. We can assess process unity by testing for similar results among the possible strata.
- How do we determine that the values we obtain come from a single causal system with *predictable* output?
- How do we know that the inputs to a process haven't somehow been altered, so that our measured output is correspondingly changed?

To answer these questions we rely on knowledge and tools from the field of statistical process control (SPC).

Control charting

A basic tool of SPC is the control chart, developed by Walter Shewhart at Western Electric (Bell Labs) in the 1920s. A control chart is a tool for:

- distinguishing signal from noise in a data set drawn from a reiterative process
- identifying when a process is predictable
- identifying when a process is not predictable.

When a process is predictable it is in a state of statistical control, and when unpredictable it is not in statistical control. A control chart presents a graphical mathematical description of the past experience with a process. Any series of data points we work with are the output of some process. When a reasonable amount of data are collected (more is always better, but 20 points is unlikely to mislead, generally at a level of at least $p = 0.01^2$), limits of expected performance are computed. If the data remain within those limits, and conform to other detection rules that may be applied (see below), then we identify a statistically stable system. Otherwise, we are dealing with a system for which we cannot make predictions. Recall now that predictability was one of the assumptions underlying our implicit approaches to filtering data. SPC thus offers an operational definition of a predictable process or system.

Control charting informs process improvement work

Our choice of methods to improve a process depends on the statistical control state of the process results. When operating in statistical control, the process is a well defined and predictably performing phenomenon. Changing the results achieved by a statistically controlled process requires re-engineering; a *new* process is required if we desire different output. Any less comprehensive type of change will not achieve the desired effect; it may actually make things worse. The current process is perfectly designed to be getting what it is getting. On the other hand, if results are not in statistical control, we begin by cleaning things up. We remove extraneous influences and make the inputs consistent. Basically, we establish what the core process we are looking at truly represents. This is the context in which responding to values representing a signal can be productive. Indeed, this may be a basis for operationally defining a measurement result that calls for a response.

Overview of creating a control chart

May I share my expository dilemma with you? If I present an illustrative control chart before explaining how to create it, I expect you will withhold credence until convinced of the technique's validity. However, if I start by explaining how to create a SPC control chart, I may bore you. So I have chosen the middle road and I ask your indulgence with the presentation. To aid your developing a functional understanding of SPC please think through the technical discussions carefully, perhaps coming back to them a second time after working with the charts.

The method for computing the control limits (to characterize whether process performance is in statistical control) reiteratively questions whether additional data points are consistent with predicted performance based on preceding data. The method begins by assuming – hypothesizing, actually – that the process whose results we are considering is performing stably over time. Assuming this, we compute a Grand Average ($\bar{X}$) and an Average Range ($m\bar{R}$) for the values. We use these computed values to obtain the control limits for the process, thereby establishing the expected amount of variation in the measured data. Subsequently obtained measurement values will either be consistent with the limits or disprove the hypothesis of statistical stability and predictability.

More specifically, we establish a lack of statistical control by identifying inconsistency between what is observed, our actual measurements, and what is expected, the computed control limits. Such inconsistency most likely indicates that the starting assumption of statistical stability is not warranted.[2]

Characterizing the variation

For a process in statistical control, the data reflect natural fluctuation – the variation inherent in the process itself. This kind of variation is called *common cause variation*. Nothing special is going on to produce any of these values. Each such data point represents a snapshot of where the process happens to be on each iteration of the process trajectory (the path it takes, what it is doing, in space-time as it creates its results). Therefore, a data set showing only common cause variation contains *no signals of significance* (to suggest that the process requires our attention or our action). Apparent variation among data points is only noise. Such a data set justifies considering that process inputs are stable and no external factors (perturbations) are altering the results. If we desire to shift the mean or tighten the control limits for a process in statistical control, we must *change the causal system*, that is, re-engineer the process – create an entirely new and predictable causal system.

For a process displaying lack of statistical control, the data reflect variation attributable to factors not inherent to the process. Explicit detection rules (presented shortly) identify data points indicating *special cause or assignable cause variation*. Special cause data points are *signals* (suggesting that the process requires our attention or our action). Reflecting either a detrimental or a beneficial effect, a special cause merits a response. If the effect is detrimental we want to eliminate it. If it is beneficial, we want to incorporate it in the process. In any case, a special cause data point is just a signal, not an answer. We must investigate why the data point occurred.

To explain special cause variation we need knowledge of the context and the process. Because the data points retain the time dimension, we investigate what went on at those times. For example, medication errors abruptly increased in July. What else happened in July? In a teaching hospital, new housestaff begin working. We test our hypothesis by studying whether the process becomes statistically controlled after removing the identified perturbation.

A clinical example: patient temperature measurement values

Berwick illustrates variation in what we measure and what we do with a data table compiled from sequential temperature measurements obtained from a patient undergoing evaluation and care for "possible osteomyelitis."[3] The patient is a 16-year-old with a clinical picture and bone scan compatible with that diagnosis, but blood cultures were negative. Despite empiric antibiotic therapy for a week, temperature spikes continued.

The fundamental clinical question was whether indeed the patient had osteomyelitis or whether there was another process operating, such as lymphoma. Berwick's temperature data are presented in Table 9.1. The original patient chart contained no such tabular compilation. Presumably, the 21 documented interventions reflect physician interpretations of the temperature data. The same data in the medical record were dispersed over 22 pages of nurses' notes.

Berwick's temperatures: XmR method

Berwick[3] used the temperature data to illustrate physicians' patterns of measuring and responsively changing care. Let's continue working with these data and create a control chart – to filter the values (that is, distinguish signal from noise) and to characterize the underlying process (that is, establish whether it is predictable or not).

We use different charts for "variables" data (continuous data), categorical data (for example, yes/no), or "counts" data (number of occurrences in some opportunity space – for example, number of occurrences of nosocomial infection per 100 patient days). For variables data, exemplified by the temperature measurements, we use an "individuals and moving range chart," referred to as an XmR chart. This chart is comprised of two time-series displays – one display showing the individual measurements (X) as they are collected over time, and a second showing the moving range (mR), a measure of the dispersion of the data.

The individual measurement values (X) are plotted as a run chart (see Chapter 7). The moving range (mR) is computed as the difference of each of two successive measurement values in the time series. From these data we may establish the SPC limits that serve as guideposts for process characterization:[2]

- For the X (individual values) chart:

  - Center line (mean) = $\bar{X}$
  - Upper control limit (in the XmR case also known as the upper natural process limit) = $\bar{X} + 2.660 m\bar{R}$
  - Lower control limit = $\bar{X} - 2.660 m\bar{R}$

- For the $m\bar{R}$ chart:

Table 9.1 Temperature data. Produced with permission from Berwick DM. *Med Care* 1991;29:1212–25[3]

Date	Temp	Action	Date	Temp	Action
16 Oct	37·1	Oxacillin		36·9	
	39·9			38·2	Tylenol
	38·5	Blood C/S; Tylenol		38·6	
	38·1			38·8	
	38·8	Tylenol		38·6	Tylenol
17 Oct	37·3			37·6	
	37·4			36·9	
	37·7		24 Oct	37·8	Tylenol
	37·5	Bone scan		36·6	
18 Oct	38·3			37·8	
	37·4			38·4	
19 Oct	39·8	Off antibiotics		38·4	Tylenol
	37·6			38·7	
	36·6			38·9	
	37·7			38·5	
	38·7	Tylenol		38·4	Tylenol
	38·7			37·8	
	39·1			36·1	
	37·8		25 Oct	36·9	Ceftazolin
	37·5			37	
20 Oct	36·5			37	Bone marrow
	36·5	Bone biopsy		37	
	36·8			38·7	
	37·1			36·2	
	36·7			37	
21 Oct	38·2		26 Oct	38·5	Tylenol
	38·2	Tylenol		37·1	
	38·4			37·3	
	37			37·5	
	38	Tylenol		36·5	
	36·9		27 Oct	36·8	
	37·7			36·1	
	37·9			37·7	
	38·7	Tylenol		38·5	
	38·8			38·5	Tylenol
	38·4			37·5	
	37·1			37	
	36·7			36·3	
	37	Tylenol	28 Oct	36·7	
22 Oct	36			36·8	
	37·2			37·3	
	38·2	Tylenol		38·8	
	38.5			37.9	

(Continued)

Table 9.1   (Continued)

Date	Temp	Action	Date	Temp	Action
	38·8			37·3	
	38·3	Tylenol	29 Oct	36·1	
	38·1			36·3	
	37·3			36·6	
	37·7	Tylenol		36·9	
23 Oct	36·1			36·9	
	36·5			37	

- Center line = $m\bar{R}$ (this is the average of the moving range values)
- Upper control limit = $3 \cdot 268 m\bar{R}$
  (Note that the moving range chart does not have a lower control limit.)
- The numbers 2·660 and 3·268 are the product of 3 dispersion units (σ) and a correction factor specific for the so-called subgroup size.

Here is one way to understand how moving ranges help to characterize the variation in the data. The moving range describes the difference between two successive results produced by the causal system under study, so these two results (presumably) were subject to the same causes.[6] This is a core concept of common cause variation – the variation "built-in" to the system. Significant trends and other markers of special cause variation are thus mR values that "stand out" against this baseline common cause variation.

We return to the XmR method in a later section, with instructions for pencil-and-paper creation of a XmR chart. Figure 9.1 shows the results of the XmR graphical method as computed using Microsoft Excel. We now are ready to discuss interpreting this graphical display.

Signal detection rules

A variety of detection rules are used to identify a signal on a SPC control chart. Although the more detection rules we

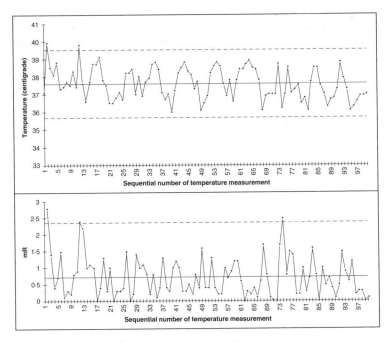

Figure 9.1   Control chart showing Berwick's temperature measurements

apply for interpreting a chart, the more likely we are to mistake noise for a signal, even when several rules are concurrently applied, false signal identification generally happens fewer than 1 time in 100.[2] The detection rule(s) you choose to employ may reflect the nature of your data – for example, you might apply rule #3 below when you observe a series of incrementing values. Commonly applied rules include:[2,5]

1   A data point lying outside of the range bounded by the upper and lower control limits.
2   Eight or more successive data points occurring on the same side of the line showing $y = \bar{X}$.
3   Seven consecutive points describing an upward or downward trend.

Signals on the moving range chart are similarly identified.

Other patterns may indicate a signal; the pattern may reflect how the data were collected or grouped, so interpretation is context-dependent (more complete discussion is available elsewhere[2,5]).

- A fourteen-point run in a sawtooth pattern. Alternating higher and lower values may result from alternately collecting data from what are really two discrete processes (recall remarks in earlier chapters about stratifying).
- Any pattern of data points that occurs repetitively may indicate even more complex aggregating of data originating in separate processes.

As an exercise, try interpreting the XmR temperature charts in the preceding section using the detection rules discussed here. Do you identify as many special cause variation points as there were interventions?

References

1 Wheeler DJ. *Understanding variation*. Knoxville, TN: SPC Press, 1993.
2 Wheeler DJ, Chambers DS. *Understanding statistical process control*. Knoxville, TN: SPC Press, 1992.
3 Berwick DM. Controlling variation in health care: a consultation from Walter Shewhart. *Med Care* 1991;**29**:1212–25.
4 Deming WE. *Out of the crisis*. Massachusetts Institute of Technology CAES, 1992.
5 Deming WE. *The new economics*. Massachusetts Institute of Technology CAES, 1994.
6 Jordan JA, Jordan LM, Ranney GB. Methods for continual improvement with applications to health care. Limited distribution; copy provided by The Center for the Evaluative Clinical Sciences at Dartmouth Medical School, 1997.

10: Understanding variation in our measurements

"But we work with human beings, not machines..."

Some readers may question applying engineering methods to living systems. The methods of control charts are rigorous and they apply to *any iterative* process, biological or not. Control charts characterize a process as predictable or not. Predictable processes are axiomatic to professional activity. If the systems we deal with are not predictable, then we have no basis for intervening.

What does a telephone manufacturing plant have in common with a hospital? (after Berwick[1])

Statistical process control began when Walter Shewhart, a physicist at the Hawthorne manufacturing plant of Bell Telephone, undertook improving the telephone production process. He discovered great variation in the way workers made adjustments to processes in response to process information. He saw this variation among individuals and even for a single individual over time. Commonly, the workers were overreacting to process information that Shewhart's SPC techniques identified as random variation – common cause variation. And when they overreacted, the variation got worse. The system became even less reliable. They were tampering. They misinterpreted noise as a signal.

How did the managers respond to this increasing variation in results and deterioration of reliability? Thinking that the processes themselves were at fault (remember, the real problem was in the way workers responded to process information), managers added corrective steps to the processes, making the processes even more complicated. The result was continued erosion of reliability and quality. (This might be a good time to refer back to Chapter 6, "Needless complexity in our care processes.")

Berwick compares this situation with decision processes in hospitals. Refer again to the temperature data in the last chapter. Using a data stream of 101 temperature measurements, six house officers and five consultants adjusted patient evaluation and care without explicit decision rules for identifying variation that "means something."[1] Look back at the XmR chart (Figure 9.1) along with the table of measurements and accompanying interventions (Table 9.1). Only three instances of special cause variation appear on the individual's portion of the XmR chart (two lie above the upper natural process limit and one is represented by a run of eight consecutive points to one side of the mean). Yet the physicians undertook so many interventions!

Might clinicians be mistaking noise for signal, signal for noise, and tampering with the system that is their patient? Responding to the question of the prevalence of tampering in medical management and resource use, Berwick says: "No one really knows. The cost could be enormous. Clinicians, flooded today with the results of measurement upon measurement, undoubtedly face serious risks of misunderstanding variation in what is being measured."[1]

SPC to help understand NICU data: an example

Summary measures alone, such as means, can hide performance information. For example, consider two NICUs, A and B, with similar monthly mean mortality rates of about 3% for a defined stratum of patients (see Figures 10.1 and 10.2). (For the point of this illustration, we will assume that the data points are justifiably aggregated.)

Unit A and Unit B have very similar mean mortality rates but the units are not performing similarly. The lower and upper control limits for Unit B are 2·4% and 3·6%; for Unit A, 1·4% and 4·6%. The control chart for NICU A tells us that the current care system, without any unusual influence, can be expected in some months to produce a mortality rate as high as 4·6%. That *would* be unusual for Unit B. Suppose the director of Unit A investigates when mortality rate more than doubles, from 1·8% to 3·9%. From what you know about SPC, is this likely to be a useful investigation? No, the effort is likely to be unproductive. On the basis of the NICU A control chart

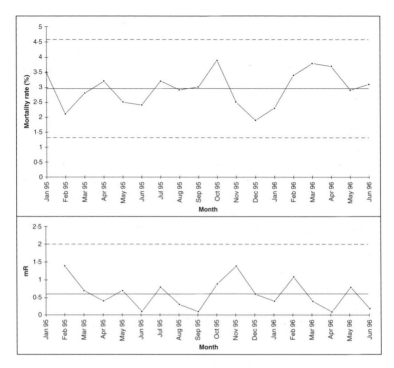

Figure 10.1 Mortality rate for NICU A

displaying a process in statistical control and the location of the upper and lower control limits for process results, we know that a change in rate from 1·8% to 3·9% can be ordinarily expected for Unit A. Here is the point: don't respond to operationally undefined "trends" and "extreme values." SPC provides operational definitions of a "trend" and of an "extreme value" – a value that "means something," a value about which we should "do something."

We remain with the issue of how to decide on the standards constituting acceptable performance. To begin, we ascertain that we are dealing with a statistically stable and well-defined process. We do this by verifying that our measurements describe only common cause variation. If instead we see evidence of special cause variation – *signals* in our data calling for investigation into the reason for the perturbation – we must first understand what happened to produce that result. We confirm that understanding when the data we collect after

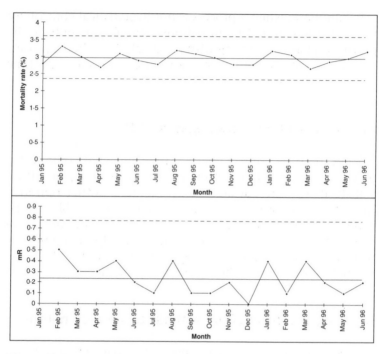

Figure 10.2 Mortality rate for NICU B

either eliminating or integrating the special cause (depending on whether the perturbing effect on process performance is unfavorable or favorable) indicate that the process is now statistically stable.

Since a process only is predictable when it is in statistical control, we must determine that this characteristic applies before we can meaningfully evaluate a process. Recognize however, that a state of statistical control has no relation to whether we will like the results we are getting. Meaningful standards for acceptable performance can be established from benchmarks and benchmarking, the subject of Chapter 11. For now, assume we incorporate these considerations in our assessment. If the process is in statistical control and we like the results we are getting, fine. If we don't like the current results and want to change them – we want different control limits and/or mean – that requires changing the entire process.

In summary: when a process is not in statistical control, we work on the external perturbations – the factors outside the process that are interfering with predictability; when a process is in statistical control but we want different results, it is time to change the process.

Computer software packages for SPC

You can create control charts using somewhat complicated macros in Microsoft Excel (as I have done here), or with a statistical software package such as Stata. Another option is Improvit, a software program designed just for SPC work. When you are comfortable with the different types of control charts and their use, this may be the most helpful and flexible program for your needs. In Chapter 14 you will find URLs for contacting these and other sources of material.

Creating a control chart without using a computer

Often the outcome measurements you make will produce a relatively small set of numbers; you can create control charts for such data using only pencil and paper. To illustrate, let's go back to the (fictional) mortality rate data used to produce the control chart for NICU A from an earlier section.

Table 10.1 reports the month and year, and the corresponding mortality rate. Recall that an XmR chart has two sub-charts: the moving range (mR), describing the dispersion of the data, and the individual values (X), showing how the data vary with time.

We work in the following sequence of steps:[2,3]

1 Use a sheet of graph paper. Divide it into two sections so that both the X and the mR data will be displayed.
2 Start by computing the moving range. Take the difference between every two X values, starting with $(X_2 - X_1)$, then $(X_3 - X_2)$, all the way through $(X_n - X_{(n-1)})$, where X_n = last X in the list. Thus, if there are n measurement values of X, there will be n–1 values of mR. For NICU A mortality rate data, n = 18, so there must be 17 data points for mR corresponding to this set.

Table 10.1 Mortality rate data used to produce the control chart from NICU A

Month	Mortality rate (%)
Jan 95	3·5
Feb 95	2·1
Mar 95	2·8
Apr 95	3·2
May 95	2·5
Jun 95	2·4
Jul 95	3·2
Aug 95	2·9
Sep 95	3·0
Oct 95	3·9
Nov 95	2·5
Dec 95	1·9
Jan 96	2·3
Feb 96	3·4
Mar 96	3·8
Apr 96	3·7
May 96	2·9
Jun 96	3·1

3 Plot the series of mR values.
4 Now compute the average mR: $\bar{R}$ = sum of mR values/ number of mR values. For the data from NICU A, $\bar{R} = 10 \cdot 4 / 17 = 0 \cdot 61176$.
5 Draw $\bar{R}$ as a solid centerline on the mR chart.
6 The upper control limit for the mR chart is computed from the formula: $UCL_{mR} = 3 \cdot 267 \times \bar{R}$. For NICU A, $UCL_{mR} = 3 \cdot 267 \times 0 \cdot 61176 = 2 \cdot 00047$.
7 Plot the UCL_{mR} on the mR chart using a dotted line. Note that when the moving range is computed from every two successive X values, a lower control limit is not computed. (Be careful that you do not consider the zero line as a lower control limit. A single point on the zero line merely describes no measured variation between two successive values (that is, zero difference between successive values). That degree of consistency does not indicate special cause variation.)
8 Some authors (Jordan *et al*[2]) identify outlier mR values and reiteratively revise $\bar{R}$ by eliminating extreme mR values. The intent is to limit inflation of the X chart limits (see below). This practice is not done by all, and for simplicity here, is omitted from the procedure.

9 Now on the X chart, plot the individual values for X.

10 Compute the average X, $\bar{X}$ = sum of the X values/number of X values. For the data from NICU A, $\bar{X}$ = 53·1/18 = 2·95.

11 Draw $\bar{X}$ as a solid centerline on the X chart.

12 Compute the upper and lower control limits (UCL$_X$, LCL$_X$) as follows: UCL$_X$ = $\bar{X}$ + 3($\bar{R}$/d$_2$) and LCL$_X$ = $\bar{X}$ − 3($\bar{R}$/d$_2$). Note that d$_2$ is the correction factor mentioned in the general discussion of control charts. In this case, where the subgroup size for mR is 2, d$_2$ as read from a table of SPC correction factors (see Wheeler) is = 1·128. (The values on this table of correction factors are computed from a mathematical model for stable variation. $\bar{R}$ gives a somewhat inflated measure of the variation among individual X values, and d$_2$ adjusts for this effect.) A similar explanation applies to the value 3·267 used for computing the mR control limit in step 6 above.

13 Plot UCL$_X$ and LCL$_X$ on the X chart using dotted lines.

(To clarify possible confusion when you read source material, rigorous discussions of XmR charting refer to control limits for X values as natural process limits.)

Evaluating control limits

Referring back to the mortality rate control charts, notice that the control limits have a narrower range for Unit B compared with Unit A – they are "tighter." Sometimes that is good. Tight control limits may indicate a superbly functioning system, one with a relatively small amount of naturally occurring variation. However, tight control limits might be telling us we are fooling ourselves with our data, that the data we are collecting are "autocorrelated."

Autocorrelation entails mistakenly using a variable as an outcome predictor when it is actually a proxy for the outcome; the variable contains much the same information that the outcome we are trying to "predict" contains. When we put the same information on both sides of a regression equation the correlation coefficient approaches a value of 1, a value you do not see in real-world systems research.

To illustrate, suppose we try to predict height from knowledge of height squared. We will gain no insight here – we're working with essentially the same information.

Restating, if we incorrectly choose to measure some variable that is not so much a predictor of our result of interest as it is another form of the same information contained in that result, the control chart will show very tight control limits. Thus, to avoid this pitfall we need good knowledge of the system context and a high degree of "process literacy" – detailed familiarity with what happens as the process unfolds.

When computing control limits we may specifically choose a level of precision to suit the evaluative context. Control limits are commonly computed using a dispersion factor of 3σ, or 3 computed dispersion units. That choice of the level of precision – the number of multiples of σ – should reflect the consequences of a mistake in signal identification. If we cannot afford to miss a signal amid the noise, we may choose to compute control limits from 2σ or rarely 1σ. If we want to minimize the likelihood of calling noise a signal, we instead might compute control limits with a higher σ multiple. For example, in managing mechanical ventilation based on measured pCO_2, if we adjust therapy when the measured change in pCO_2 represents only noise (but we thought it was a signal), we are *tampering*. So we might (after also considering other factors relevant to pCO_2 and the patient's well-being) apply a relatively higher σ multiple in characterizing such a run of data points.

Analytic statistics, enumerative statistics, and comparing results among NICUs

In discussing measurement (Chapter 8), I indicated that when studying a *single* system we do not need to risk adjust before making inference from the data, provided the data are in statistical control. So when making inference from a single system we ask whether the causal system is well defined and predictable. When comparing *two or more* systems, we ask different questions:

1 Do the data we are looking at come from the same system or process?
2 Do the data we are looking at come from the same population?

We use a different line of statistical reasoning to answer questions about system or process performance than we use to answer questions of population origin for a sample. When thinking about the population origin of sampled data, the appropriate theoretical model is *enumerative statistics*. This is the statistical approach readers more likely are already familiar with, involving such techniques of hypothesis testing as the t-test and analysis of variance (ANOVA). When thinking about the process that generated the data set, the appropriate theoretical model is *analytic statistics*. Exemplified by techniques of statistical process control, analytic statistical reasoning informs us whether the data are likely to be coming from a predictable and well-defined causal system. The data comparison we make here is historical. We want to know whether more recently obtained measurements are consistent with what the system produced before, asking: Does this system we are studying seem to be operating now as it has been in the past – are the results predictable? If our answer is no, if the data are not in statistical control, then we know that inputs and/or processes are not constant.

Before comparing performance among NICUs we risk adjust the data, accounting for known differences in care processes and inputs that can affect the corresponding measured end-results. It should now be clear that if the data we wish to compare are resulting from reiterative processes unfolding over time, we must also establish that the data are coming from respective systems that are each in statistical control. Comparing data sets resulting from unpredictable processes is not meaningful.

Recapping

What is actual is actual only for one time.
And only for one place.

TS Eliot

From the stream of data produced by the reiterative processes we study, our task is to distinguish – explicitly, and by using valid decision rules – which events are signals, which are noise.

References

1 Berwick DM. Controlling variation in health care: a consultation from Walter Shewhart. *Med Care* 1991;**29**:1212–25.
2 Jordan JA, Jordan LM, Ranney GB. *Methods for continual improvement with applications to health care.* Limited distribution; copy provided by The Center for the Evaluative Clinical Sciences at Dartmouth Medical School, 1997.
3 Block P. *Flawless consulting.* San Francisco, CA: Pfeiffer & Company, 1981.

Part 3:
Action

Knowing is not enough, we must apply. Willing is not enough, we must do.

Johann Goethe

11: Benchmarks and benchmarking

There is always one best result and one best process for achieving that result ... And they can always be improved.

B Joiner

Definitions

A *benchmark* is a statistical measure against which to make a comparison. *Benchmarking* entails measuring what you do against what others you respect are doing. The task is finding the "best practices." Benchmarking is a *systematic* process, a *method* for finding "the best of the best." Thinking this way leads us outside our usual frame of reference. Identifying a gap between what you do and what someone else with better results is doing creates tension for change, encouraging action.

A benchmarking story

Max DePree tells an apropos story:[1]

A German company making machine tools succeeded in creating a long-sought-after drill bit. This bit could drill a hole the diameter of a human hair through a thick plate of hardened steel. Understandably, the Germans were rather excited about their accomplishment and sent off samples to colleagues and potential customers in Russia, the United States, and Japan. They anticipated congratulations and sales orders.

The Russians never responded.

The Americans wanted to know about unit pricing, special contractual purchasing arrangements, and licensing rights to produce the bit in their own factories.

Several months went by before hearing from the Japanese. Their reply was polite, apologizing for the delay in extending their congratulations on the achievement. Continuing, they said the original bit was enclosed, now with a slight modification to it. The Germans looked at their almost invisibly thin drill bit, noticing nothing different. So they examined it under the microscope. To their amazement, the Japanese had drilled an even smaller-bore hole right down the center of the German bit!

Do we work in neonatology as the Japanese are portrayed here? I think not. The Japanese work perspective in the story employs benchmarks and benchmarking to drive breakthrough achievement. A "breakthrough" is a qualitatively new way of doing something that achieves previously unheard-of results. The computer industry has seen a great deal of breakthrough activity over the past few decades. I remember paying over $1000 for a 128K machine 17 years ago. Now my pocket memo/organizer device has more memory than that, and it cost about $30.

Can you imagine achieving substantially improved NICU outcomes at significantly lower cost than we currently do? That we haven't seems not for lack of trying. Increasingly, professional colleagues relate working harder, trying harder to achieve the best results they can. No, effort is not the central issue; rather, it's *how* we are trying to improve our work and the results we achieve.

The limitations of local knowledge

We need to incorporate benchmarking and benchmarks in our work because an exclusively local knowledge base constrains our thinking. Recall from Chapter 1 the discussion of system boundaries and evaluative perspective. When we are close to our experience we may not see the patterns among the events that might be evident from a distance. Objectivity, a view from outside the system, may disclose such patterns at the price of within-system information loss. Each perspective contributes to our understanding. Against this background, let's consider some of the barriers to improving our care – and at the same time, reasons to incorporate benchmarking and benchmarks in our daily work.[2]

- *We usually don't watch our colleagues as they work.* The core unit of health care activity is often the patient and her (his) physician. Thought processes and care processes are not evident to others (and perhaps sometimes at all). The point is that we are not used to benchmarking – it has not been an integral part of the way we practice medicine and provide care.

- *We lack detailed information about how we implement our knowledge of health care.* This prevents our understanding "the fine structure of care and makes studies linking practices to outcomes difficult."[2] From our experience in training and in independent practice, we are familiar with the individualized style of practice among physicians. During my neonatology fellowship, every Monday morning that the attending physicians changed responsibility for NICU coverage, I ran around for a couple of hours changing countless aspects of care to conform to the preferences of the attending physician coming on service. While the faculty was amused by this behavior (displayed by most fellowship trainees), they did not appear to reflect on its significance. Often we do not know enough about what our colleagues do either to scrutinize it or to generalize about it. Yet physicians seem to commonly spurn guidelines for care that are intended to decrease unintended variation. If individualized approaches to practice are better, we must be able to demonstrate that to be the case. So far, support is lacking.[3]

- *Because we are not yet well organized to compare our processes of care or their results, we cannot know with much certainty the quality of care we are providing.* Now there are efforts underway to change this. The Institute for Healthcare Improvement, in Boston, does much good work in this area (http://www.ihi.org). The Vermont Oxford Database identifies "substantial variation among individual NICUs" in outcomes and resource use.[4] These findings, in part, drive the NIC/Q and NIC/Q 2000 benchmarking and quality improvement collaboratives of that network.[4]

- *Adverse outcomes typically occur infrequently so the volume of such local experience tends to remain low.* An individual institution may simply not have enough experience to understand some causal sequences. Consider the last 100 infants under 28 weeks gestation that you cared for. Suppose four of them died: one from air-block syndrome, one from septic shock, one from NEC, and one from intraventricular hemorrhage. These deaths do not constitute a sufficient experience base for developing informed and beneficial changes in the current care practices. There is not enough information contained by those four terminal cases from which to derive a predictive model of risk. How different it would be if we were working with data from hundreds or thousands of such cases, and if the care processes involved were explicit and detailed! Having said this, remember that the bulk of the results you are always working to improve are not rare occurrences. Good work in these areas can be done locally. The point is that improvement work can operate at more than the one organizational level. The unit of analysis depends on a requisite volume of experience for the selected process or outcome.

• *Hospitals and clinicians reject "quality improvement" efforts that lay blame instead of inform motivated professionals with constructive change ideas. "... frightening physicians to higher levels of performance is absurd."*[2]

Benchmarking does improve health care outcomes

The Northern New England Cardiovascular Disease Study Group (NNECVDSG) demonstrated that results of coronary artery bypass graft (CABG) surgery substantially improved while processes became significantly streamlined as a result of a multi-center collaborative benchmarking and continual improvement effort.[5] These authors enumerate 18 changes in processes of CABG surgery as a result of benchmarking site visits among the participating centers. The group used a logistic regression model for expected mortality to risk adjust among centers and to evaluate the effect of the process improvement intervention (that is, they compared observed with expected outcomes). Post-intervention, expected mortality declined 24% (p = 0·001). Importantly, the authors couldn't attribute the results to particular changes. Rather, they invoked the Japanese concept of *kaizen* – "doing things better, little by little, all the time."[5] (Think back to our discussion of the *muda* of needless complexity in Chapter 6.)

Preliminary analysis of the Vermont Oxford Network NIC/Q Project, working similarly to the NNECVDSG, indicates reduction in nosocomial infection and chronic lung disease for a defined cohort of patients.[6]

Benchmarking as "real time science"

Critics question whether a benchmarking collaborative like the NNECVDSG represents science.[7] Berwick calls it a special kind of science – "real time science."[7] Continuing, he says that when the aim is to learn about the fine details of improving a process, randomized trials appear to be far less efficient than the techniques used by the NNECVDSG (substantially the same as the approach in the present book).

Learning about process fine structure, identifying leverage points, and generating improvement ideas benefit from front-line involvement in care and real-time observation. But the knowledge is often institution-specific, not generalizable. Recall that the NNECVDSG workers reported inability to attribute their improvements to particular changes, instead referring to *kaizen* – "doing things better, little by little, all the time."[5] Most likely, what was done to improve end-results differed among each hospital and each surgeon. "One surgeon learned from another's interesting approach to hemostasis, while the second studied the first's rehabilitation plans ..."[7] Let us be careful to distinguish this kind of work from some workers' accusations of a haphazard, trial-and-error approach. It is nothing of the kind. Reflect on all you have read about improvement work in this book. This type of work represents "careful, inductive learning by experts who have deep knowledge of their own work."[7]

Benchmarking for improving our work and meeting our patients' expectations

Patients are entitled to know what to expect, quantitatively and accurately, when they interact with a health care system;

they want to know "their chances." Physicians need to know how they are doing, quantitatively and accurately.

This book is an invitation to understand the fine structure of problems many of us may not have even known existed in our practice of medicine. They are problems that are intractable by the methods most of us acquired during formal medical education and in our subsequent experience. If they were otherwise, would they still be with us? The problems require more than just new knowledge and tools. They require the combined efforts of larger groups of people than perhaps we are accustomed to working in. They require assessments that go outside our usual frame of reference. Too often in the past few years, physicians have banded together to deal with the changes going on in the health care environment, but with unclear aims. *Inter-institutional collaboration is a prerequisite for comprehensive health care information mastery.*

Another category of *muda*

We may add another category of *muda* to our already lengthy enumeration in Chapter 2. Providing health care in an environment of *unexamined* variation entails *muda*. We know that variation occurs wherever we look, and we assume that no one prefers results less good than the best. Therefore, when we fail to regularly characterize the results we achieve, when we fail to compare them to benchmarks, and fail to include benchmarking activities as a part of our work, we necessarily harbor *muda* in our work.

John Wennberg's key questions for health care

Alas, examining the variation in care and results among our NICUs and working to decrease it does not necessarily eliminate *muda*. Another aspect of decreasing *muda* calls for us to distinguish assumption from established knowledge. For example, 21 per cent of births in the United States in 1995 were cesarean deliveries. The Department of Health and Human Services has established a goal of a 15 per cent cesarean delivery rate for the year 2000. Clear data substantiating the safety and overall desirability of this rate do not exist.[8]

John Wennberg first called the scientific community's attention to practice variation more than twenty-five years ago.[9] As we examine our data and compare our results with those of our colleagues, we may guide our overall assessment and our efforts to reduce *muda* by three fundamental and overarching questions that Wennberg poses:[3]

1 "Which rate is right?"
2 "How much [care] is enough?" Do you assume that more health care is always better than less? From a systems perspective, "more" of something typically means more system interconnections as well. Recall from Chapter 6 how more interconnections (complexity) may adversely affect quality, reliability and predictability. You may now better appreciate the extent to which confounding plays a role in our studies to answer the question of whether "more is better."
3 " What is fair?" This question is related to the notion of the "tragedy of the commons," articulated thirty years ago by Garret Hardin.[10] When individuals overuse finite and shared resources for their short-term benefit, the communal benefits progressively diminish.

Parents and caregivers often speak of "doing everything" for a complexly ill patient. From either an individual or a community standpoint, is this meaningful?

References

1 DePree M. *Leadership jazz*. New York: Dell Trade Paperbacks, 1992.
2 O'Connor GT, Plume SK, Wennberg JE. Regional organization for outcomes research. *Ann N Y Acad Sci* 1993;**703**:44–51.
3 Wennberg JE, ed. The Center for the Evaluative Clinical Sciences, DMS. *The Dartmouth atlas of health care in the United States*. Chicago, IL: American Hospital Publishing, 1998.
4 Horbar JD. *A national evidence-based quality improvement collaborative for neonatology, Vermont Oxford Network, 1997, Annual Network Update*. Washington, DC, December 7, 1997.
5 O'Connor GT, Plume SK, Olmstead EM, *et al.* ftNNECDSG. A regional intervention to improve the hospital mortality associated with coronary bypass graft surgery. *JAMA* 1996;**275**:841–6.
6 Horbar J, Rogowski J, Plsek P. Project eaFtVONNQ. Collaborative quality improvement for neonatal intensive care. *Pediatr Res* 1998;**43**:177A (abstract).

7   Berwick DM. Harvesting knowledge from improvement. *JAMA* 1996; **275**:877–8.

8   Sachs BP, Kobelin C, Castro MA, Frigoletto F. The risks of lowering the cesarean-delivery rate. *N Engl J Med* 1999;**340**:54–7.

9   Wennberg J, Gittelsohn. Small area variations in health care delivery. *Science* 1973;**182**:1102–8.

10 Hardin G. The tragedy of the commons. *Science* 1968;**162**:1243–8.

12: Keeping track of what you decided to measure

At the moment of truth, there are either reasons or results.

Chuck Yaeger

An instrument panel display: what and why

Now that we've identified what to measure and collected the data, we next want to facilitate team members' understanding of it and to encourage their using it. All too often, well-intentioned and highly motivated people proudly present their results in a thick document of tables and charts. "Look at all we've done," they might say. They think the document is impressive, while the recipients of this gift, overwhelmed by the sheer quantity of information, cannot act on it. A better reporting approach entails creating an "instrument panel" display of only the most important results needed to inform an evidence-based response. Don't let the word "important" in the last sentence slip right by; have your group operationally define what they will consider an important variable to report.

When we look outside the health care field, professionals with decision and oversight responsibility for a complex system typically rely on an instrument panel to inform them how things are going. Consider, for example, operating a jet plane.[1] We take for granted that pilots use the instrument panel to guide their flight decisions. Wouldn't it be strange if they had to climb out on the wings to gather information about flap position and airspeed, go down into the fuel tanks to check the level, open the window to get atmospheric data, etc? Now think about the information gathering process in the NICU. Can your unit benefit from organizing the data that is important and displaying it graphically in a way that facilitates understanding of what is going on?

Configuring an instrument panel display of how we're doing in the NICU

When I speak with NICU workers about these ideas, they commonly get stuck on the notion that we need to create some slick software that will give us a NICU instrument panel. When *comprehensive* electronic medical records have become the standard, some type of standardized software approach might work. Until then, because of the diversity of information sources and analytic choices, an automated approach might not produce the desired results.

Your instrument panel displays the data informing you about the specific processes and results that your unit has chosen to understand better and to improve. To encourage complete and thoughtful scrutiny of the data by team members, try limiting the display to one side of one sheet of paper. Obviously, much information may thus not be displayed. But the "one side/one sheet" constraint focuses our thinking. Also, avoid presenting tabular data. A well-designed graph will render the same information more accessible.[2,3]

The composition of the NICU instrument panel is fluid. When we continually learn, that means we continually learn about different things. Instrument panel displays will vary among NICUs and also over time within a single NICU. The information display is a function of the current questions.

A checklist for creating an instrument panel display of process performance

Here is a checklist of considerations, adapted from Nelson *et al*, to help with creating an NICU instrument panel display of the core information related to your improvement efforts.[4]

To prepare an instrument panel display

* *Identify the outcomes.* Write an explicit statement of what you want to measure.
* Describe in writing, as explicitly as possible, how studying the identified outcomes will help to understand what is being done in your NICU. Specifically address:

- Exactly what is the question we seek to answer? What are we really trying to understand?
- What data will we need to answer the question?
- Create operational definitions for what you will measure – that is, the variables, the outcomes, you will study.
- *Think about how you will group the data.* Do you risk obscuring information by aggregating things that shouldn't be? Might we see important differences among groups if we stratified our data to reflect the differences among the subjects involved in the outcome we are studying?
- *Assign ownership in the process.* Who will collect the data? What sources must the data collector review to get the information?
- Develop a process for checking accuracy and completeness of the collected data.
    - Write it out: "Collected data will be considered *accurate* after the following are verified:
        - (a) _____
        - (b) _____
        - (c) _____ "

        "Collected data will be considered *complete* after the following are verified:
        - (d) _____
        - (e) _____
        - (f) _____ "
    - Ensure that you operationally defined the terms that filled in the blanks.
- Make the measuring and data collecting activities a part of the daily work of the NICU.
    - We tend to distinguish the "daily routine" from uninvited extra work. The activities discussed in this book are not "additional work." They are a basic part of thoughtful and productive daily work. The time for concern about doing "extra" work is precisely when we *don't* understand our work in detail.
- *Decide how to display the data.*
    - For example, benchmark data might be displayed on a "radar" chart showing the respective values for your

NICU and "the best of the best", for each outcome selected for the instrument panel.[5] General prescriptions will limit your thinking, but consider your outcomes and decide how to display the data so that:

(a) You preserve as much information as possible.
(b) You can easily appreciate relationships among data.
(c) The data arrangement facilitates broad understanding of the information contained in the overall data set.
(d) The displayed data supports decisions for subsequent action.

- Options that satisfy these considerations include:
  - *Control charts.* Verify that the type of chart is appropriate for the data:

    (a) *XmR charts* for "individuals" data (continuous variables).
    (b) *p-charts and np-charts* for representing the proportion of a subgroup classified into one of two categories (dichotomous data, such as disease/no disease or survived/died).
    (c) *u-charts and c-charts* for counts of an outcome of interest per "area of opportunity" (for example, infections per 1000 patient days).[2]

- Run charts.
- Histograms.
- Scatter plots.
- Pareto charts.

Don't be afraid to be innovative in your data display; if they are consonant with the purpose of the investigation, new ways of looking at the data may be just what you need to facilitate new insight.[3]

- Verify that the collected data answer the question.

An example of a first-iteration display

Here is an illustration of one way to get started. This is a list of the displays chosen by a team I recently worked with:

1 Pareto chart showing the ranking of the things we do well (staff survey).

2 Pareto chart showing the ranking of the things we could do better (staff survey).

3 XmR control chart showing the time for admitting a patient (operationally defined).

4 XmR control chart showing the time for feeding an infant (operationally defined).

5 U-chart (SPC control chart) showing, by month, the number of nosocomial infection episodes per 100 patient days of exposure, for a two year period.

6 Benchmark data for 3, 4, and 5. Radar chart (a multiple axis method for comparing two or more arrays of data – a standard option in Microsoft Excel) showing each variable.

Authentic improvement work requires a safe environment, one where workers need not fear the information collected.[6] Deming's expression for this idea was to "drive out fear" from the workplace.[6,7] When people feel safe, when they feel that the investigation is directed to *authentically* improving what is done rather than trying to put someone in the "hot seat", they become invaluable contributors to the process. This is why the data in the illustration of one team's approach to developing an instrument panel (see Figure 12.1) must be fictional.

Relating the checklist for guiding instrument panel creation with the illustrative display

Let's reconcile the instrument panel checklist with the illustrative panel.

The panel components describe the outcome variables and the method of display.

Here is a possible statement describing how the chosen outcomes will help to understand what is being done in the NICU:

On this first attempt at systematically understanding and improving our work in the NICU, we want to begin to learn about where to focus our attention, what to measure and how to measure. We want to start simply, to work with activities we think we know well.

The specific questions we want to answer are:

1 What things are we doing well?

2 What things could we do better?

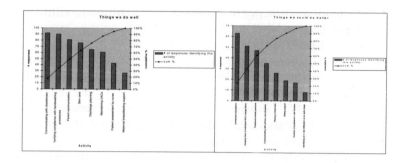

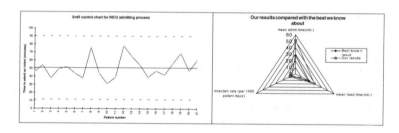

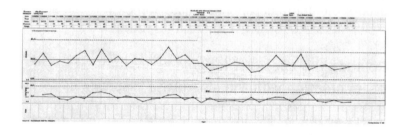

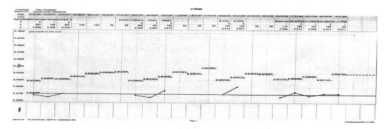

Figure 12.1   Sample NICU instrument panel display

3 Are we using our staff resources well when we admit an infant to the NICU? (We operationally define "well" in terms of process time.)

4 Are we using our staff resources well when a nurse feeds an infant in the NICU? (We operationally define "well" in terms of process time.)

5 When does a change in our nosocomial infection rate constitute a signal that merits our response?

6 Are the mean rate and the upper and lower control limit values acceptable (see 7, below)? What results merit a response?

7 How are we doing with 3, 4, and 5 compared with the best results we know of at other NICUs?

Accuracy and completeness

The time for admitting an infant and the time for feeding an infant are verified by the nurse performing the process. She documents in a nursing addendum the operationally defined components of the task. This approach reflects an attempt to make the initiative a part of the daily work.

Here are operational definitions for outcome measurement:

1 The procedure of admitting a patient to the NICU *begins* when the infant arrives at the NICU door and *ends* when the nursing admission assessment sheet is completed and the nurse has reviewed the physician's admitting orders.

2 The procedure of feeding an infant *begins* with taking vital signs and changing the diaper, bed linen, and clothes, if needed, and *ends* after charting the care episode.

3 Nosocomial infection is defined as described in CDC guidelines on file with the infection control nurse. The count of patient days appears in the NICU census log.

Let's also reconcile the display panel with Langley and co-workers' overarching questions for improvement work:[8]

• *What are we trying to accomplish?* We want to improve the quality of our care. We hope to improve our work and the associated outcomes by making activities that increase our understanding of our work a part of our daily routine. We know that this is a reiterative activity that never ends. In particular, we want to decrease the time a nurse needs to admit an infant and to feed an infant. We want to promptly and accurately distinguish noise and signal in nosocomial infection data.

- *What change can we make that will result in an improvement?* For admitting and feeding an infant, we will draw change ideas from our study of the process maps we create. Change ideas regarding nosocomial infection rate will come from a cause and effect diagram and related process map created by the team.

- How will we know that a change is an improvement? For:

  - *Things we do well*: New items will appear on the Pareto chart and previously appearing items will persist.
  - *Things we can do better*: Items will not recurrently appear on this chart with subsequent iterations of the improvement effort.
  - *Time for admitting a patient*: The mean will decrease and the control limits will become tighter.
  - *Time for nurse feeding of a patient*: The mean will decrease and the control limits will become tighter.
  - *Numbers of nosocomial infections per 100 patient days*: The data will be in statistical control, the mean will decrease, and the upper control limit will decrease. The frequency of outbreaks of infection with the same organism for greater than one month in succession will diminish.

- *Benchmark data*: We want to exceed the best reported results we know of.

I expect thoughtful readers may not agree with some of the data choices for the illustrative instrument panel. You might ask, for example, whether items 1 and 2, "things we do well" and "things we could do better" are tautologically recursive in the context of an instrument panel. These items also lack operational definitions. As for measuring the time for feeding an infant, isn't that just a function of an infant's care needs?

Absolute judgments of correct and incorrect for an instrument panel display miss the point of the activity. The panel configuration changes with time because the accumulating information drives continuous learning. The illustrative panel is a *first iteration* attempt. The effort accomplishes its aim if subsequent review leads to more exactly expressed questions and clearer understanding of the system. Getting started on work that will be critically revised as experience accumulates may be preferable to getting bogged down with trying to create a benchmark product on the first attempt.

The best is the enemy of the good.

Voltaire

Here are two illustrations of practical benefits for prioritizing continual thoughtfulness above first-iteration perfection:

- "Things we do well" and "Things we could do better" might be more carefully looked at in subsequent iterations. After operationally defining each item on the survey, the team can collect data for each item. They can then compare "observed v expected" – that is, how the team thinks they are doing with the actual measured performance. The exercise can be illuminating and motivating. What began as inadequately crafted ideas becomes a wake-up call to the complacent (see Chapter 13).
- "Time for feeding an infant" might be informative in relation to the chosen unit of analysis. For example, if the unit of analysis is an individual infant, XmR control chart data points would describe a multitude of different processes – disease processes, care processes, indeed anything at all associated with an infant in the context of feeding. Lumping data this way may obscure learning. However, choose nursing shift as the unit of analysis and you discover something interesting in the data. The mean feeding time during the night shift is eight minutes lower than the mean during the day shift and the night shift control limits are tighter. You have discovered that the feeding process at night is somehow different. You will want to learn more about this, because if infants are fed every three hours, and if the day shift used the night feeding process, four feedings a day would each require eight fewer minutes. This alone would save 53.3 staff hours per 100 patient days.

References

1 Nelson EC, Batalden PB, Plume SK, *et al.* Report cards or instrument panels: who needs what? *The Joint Commission Journal on Quality Improvement* 1995;**21**:155–66.
2 Wheeler DJ. *Understanding variation.* Knoxville, TN: SPC Press, 1993.
3 Tufte ER. *The visual display of quantitative information.* Cheshire, CT: Graphics Press, 1983.
4 Nelson EC, Splaine ME, Batalden PB, *et al.* Building measurement and data collection into medical practice. *Ann Intern Med* 1998;**128**:460–6.
5 Brassard M, Ritter D. *The memory jogger II.* Methuen, MA: GOAL/QPC, 1994.
6 Deming WE. *Out of the crisis.* Massachusetts Institute of Technology CAES, 1992.
7 Deming WE. *The new economics.* Massachusetts Institute of Technology CAES, 1994.
8 Langley GJ, Nolan KM, Nolan TW, *et al. The improvement guide.* San Francisco, CA: Jossey-Bass, 1996.

13: Change and people

Tell me, I may listen. Teach me, I may remember.
Involve me, I may do it.

Chinese proverb

Another component of improvement work: implementing ideas

Do you respond with trepidation to an announcement of impending organizational change? People working within a system know that positive change requires deep and comprehensive knowledge of that system; otherwise things usually get worse. So when the change doesn't come from people who *really* know how things work, we worry about the results. But even when the change ideas come from the "front line," we must also know how to *implement* that change properly.

While even initial high level views of a system may appear rather complicated, in turning ideas into action we discover and work with progressively greater levels of detail and interconnection. The detail and interconnection remaining for our examination is a pivotal component for understanding our work systems – *people*.

People underlie improvement work

Earlier, we discussed efficacy and efficiency as functions of how we implement knowledge of pathophysiology and therapeutics. Now let's look at the substrate and context for our knowledge implementation – the modality for turning our ideas into action. That modality, obvious but sometimes forgotten, is *people*. People as systems, not as objects. I suggest we begin with this assumption: before people will be interested in doing their work well and then in doing it even better, they must care about their work.

Motivating people at work

Treat people as if they were what they ought to be, and you help them become what they are capable of being.

Johann Goethe

Frederick Herzberg wrote what has become a classic article on motivating people at work.[1] He distinguishes between the things at work producing job satisfaction and motivation, and the things producing job dissatisfaction. You might think that the feelings of job satisfaction and job dissatisfaction are simply opposites of each other. Although the words themselves suggest this, psychological studies, replicated in a wide variety of populations and cultures, indicate otherwise. "The opposite of job satisfaction is not job dissatisfaction, but, rather, *no* job satisfaction; and similarly, the opposite of job dissatisfaction is not job satisfaction, but *no* job dissatisfaction."[1] This resonates with the view that considers the opposite of love to be not hate, but apathy.

Herzberg thinks about work as satisfying two sets of basic human needs. For our need for food, shelter, physical comfort, and minimizing pain, we must earn money. But we have other needs too. We want to achieve what we set out to do. When we succeed in achieving our goals we experience psychological growth. At work, the challenges from which we grow represent the *job content*; the remaining job stimuli represent the *job environment*.

Herzberg categorizes two sets of psychological factors, each set congruent with a respective set of basic human needs: growth or motivator factors, and dissatisfaction-avoidance or hygiene factors. Study after study finds the motivators explain job satisfaction and the hygiene factors explain job dissatisfaction. Reiterating, job feelings are not explained by the presence or absence of the *same* set of factors. Each feeling category, that is, satisfaction or dissatisfaction, is associated with one of two mutually exclusive sets of factors. Table 13.1 (adapted from Herzberg[1]) summarizes the findings in descending frequency of occurrence.

Table 13.1 Psychological factors. Adapted from Herzberg F. *Harvard Business Review* 1987:109–20[1]	
Job factors leading to extreme dissatisfaction	**Job factors leading to extreme satisfaction**
Company policy and administration	Achievement
Supervision	Recognition
Relationship with supervisor	Work itself
Work conditions	Responsibility
Salary	Advancement
Relationship with peers	Growth
Personal life	
Relationship with subordinates	
Status	
Security	

Motivational job characteristics

Obvious as it seems, the way to encourage intrinsic motivation in workers is to offer satisfying work.

We want to match the job challenges with a person's skills. This condition enables "flow," "the state in which people are so involved in an activity that nothing else seems to matter."[2] When our skills exceed the challenges before us, we are bored. On the other hand, when the challenges overshadow the requisite skills we feel anxiety. In this model, work can be increasingly absorbing and enjoyable when the challenges and the requisite skills increase in a coordinated manner.

This model also offers a reasonable approach to promotion and leadership: identify those people whose skills overshadow the challenges presented to them.

Tying it all together

Recalling our discussion of blame in Chapter 1, we commonly have a choice when establishing a job within our system:

We can try to work around system design deficiencies by hiring an extraordinary individual.

We can design the system and the job so that an ordinary individual (properly qualified, of course) can do the job well.

Of the two, which do you think entails less *muda* and results in improved measures of efficacy and efficiency?

Leader and change agent: core roles for improvement work

Everyone thinks of changing the world, but no one thinks of changing himself.

Leo Tolstoy

When you apply the content of this book to your work, you take on at least two roles: *leader* and *change agent*. The following material invites you to consider leadership and change from many perspectives, not just the leader's: the followers, the service recipients, the system aims, and any other appropriate perspective that comes to mind.

Implementing change

Whether or not we support a solution depends a lot on whether it's being done to us – or by us.

Sam Horn

John Kotter writes about conditions that facilitate leading organizational change.[3] The following bullet points distill his insights and frame them for the NICU context.

- *Establish a sense of urgency.* Authors also refer to this as "creating a burning platform" (off which the "changee" must jump). Make it clear why things must change.
  - Be honest about the current reality the NICU faces. Avoid "happy talk" that covers up problems calling for attention. Consider whether current performance measures tell the story that most closely resonates with the aims of the NICU.
  - Clearly lay out the future opportunities for the NICU, the rewards that may come to individuals and the group, and why as things stand now, those opportunities cannot be pursued.

- Target complacency. NICU staff can never justifiably say: "we're doing well enough."
- *Develop a vision and strategy* (refer also to the section on vision in Chapter 2). Create a verbal picture of the way the NICU will look in the future. Make it something that:
  - stakeholders can easily imagine
  - appeals to them
  - is realistic, attainable
  - is sufficiently detailed to guide decisions
  - is sufficiently flexible to allow individual expression and adaptation to unforeseen contingencies.
- *Generate short-term wins.* People are often impatient. Sustaining a great idea requiring two years to prove itself is very difficult. Break it up; along the way:
  - show that in the short run, sacrifices are justified
  - make it possible to fine-tune the efforts
  - deprive the cynics their nay-saying by providing stepwise evidence
  - build momentum.
- *Anchor new approaches in the culture.* Don't try to change the norms and values of a group early in the organizational change. The existing culture is comprised of the solutions that have already been demonstrated to work. So first demonstrate how the new solution works. Facilitate trials of the new ways, show the results, and show the connection between new ways and methods and the new, better results.

Some of these points should sound familiar. They have already appeared elsewhere in this guide, in somewhat different contexts. This is how it is with systems.

Factors accounting for the spread and acceptance of new ideas

Personalities and innovation

Be not the first by whom the new is tried,
Nor the last to lay the old aside.

Alexander Pope

Now that we've looked at an organizationally framed approach to implementing change, let's drill down and look at how individuals vary in their receptivity and their responses to new ideas. Organizational sociologists and psychologists call this studying the diffusion of innovations. My experience working in NICUs supports Rogers' way of classifying members of a group on the basis of their receptivity to new ideas.[4]

- *Innovators.* These people are "venturesome." Their social circles extend outside the local community. Innovators keep in touch with each other, even over great distances. Innovators are:
  - comfortable dealing with uncertainty
  - facile with complex technical knowledge
  - financially able to tolerate an idea that fails.
- *Early adopters.* Their social context is more local than the innovators. They are opinion leaders. These people tend to be:
  - respected by their peers
  - judicious in their behavior
  - successful in their choices. Therefore, early adopters are seen as the people "to check with" when something new is being considered. *These are the people to seek out for speeding up adopting a change.*
- *Early majority.* This is the group following Pope's advice quoted at the start of this section. Although involved with their peers, they are not leaders. According to Rogers, about one-third of the people in a group fit this category.
- *Late majority.* These people make up another third of the total in a group. Steered by financial or peer pressure or both, they adopt an innovation later than average. The risk associated with adopting a new idea looms large for this group. They are the skeptics in the group at large.
- *Laggards.* These people are the last to adopt a new idea among the group. They tend to be anchored in the past. Socially, their focus is the most local of all the categories. They tend to be suspicious of change, keeping with people thinking similarly. It takes a long time for these people to accept something new. Rogers points out the unfair negative connotation often associated with the word for

this category. Unfair, because we often attach a value judgment to the term. We may be better served in dealing with this category by not thinking in terms of the individual's shortcomings. Try instead to frame the notion of a laggard as reflecting a shortcoming of the system the laggard is in.

Tactics for engaging people with an innovation

This categorical scheme offers a useful way to approach changing a system: adjust your tactics according to the individual you wish to engage. Understanding how people vary in their receptivity to new ideas facilitates getting a new idea *accepted* rather than imposing it by forced compliance. The latter demands that a system perform beyond its capability – outside the control limits. Demanding compliance leads people to distort either the data or the system. When you work with knowledge of the factors facilitating the diffusion of innovations you can thoughtfully re-engineer, if you will, the system that is the group of people being asked to change.

Therefore, don't focus on the laggards early in your efforts to change something in the NICU. The high leverage sub-group is the early adopters. Focusing on this third of the group will require relatively less personal effort and resource use but will likely yield disproportionately great progress toward the goal.

Recognize as well, that resistance to change is only one side of the coin; the other side represents system stability. For a system to persist over time, to be resilient and robust in the face of changing circumstances, mechanisms are operating to protect system integrity. What appears to a change agent as resistance to change may be a system devotee's well-intentioned (but perhaps shortsighted) effort to preserve stability.

You will want specifically to choose the media and the communicator for presenting an improvement project to the group. Face to face communication by early adopter "near peers" sharing their subjective evaluation works well. In other words, early adopters are receptive to in-person persuasion by other already convinced early adopters. A shared knowledge base, homophily, promotes credibility for the change agent.

Heterophily has the opposite effect; thus the suggestion to rely on "near peer" communicators. More concretely, neonatologists, rather than other types of professionals, may be more effective persuaders of other neonatologists.

Criteria for acceptability of an innovation

Here are some factors that may underlie how quickly an innovation is accepted:[4]

1 Relative advantage of the innovation compared with the previous approach.
2 Compatibility of the innovation with what is currently done.
3 Complexity – how difficult is the new idea to understand and use?
4 Trialability – how easily can the idea be tested?
5 Observability – how easily can others see what has been done?

Even what we *call* an innovation can affect its perceived compatibility and therefore its rate of adoption. For example, I often notice a glazed look come over physicians' faces when acronyms containing the letter "Q," such as "QI," "TQM," and "CQI," are used in discussion during hospital committee meetings. Call it a variant of outcomes research instead, and attention levels rise as pupillary diameter increases (well, perhaps I'm exaggerating a bit here).

Conceptual drift: re-invention

Sometimes an innovation is accepted, but it becomes more or less insidiously altered into something that may or may not be an improvement on the original. "Re-invention" occurs because:[4]

- the idea is too complex – the idea is not user-friendly; it is too difficult to understand or to use
- users lack full knowledge of the innovation – this point highlights the importance of content, style, and media choice for effectively communicating
- the innovation is still only an abstract concept; it was promoted before it was adequately developed

- the innovation was implemented to solve a wide range of user problems; this is the benchmarking problem viewed from a fresh perspective: a given solution works differently in each setting
- local pride.

Greg Blonder relates an interesting story of reinvention.[5] In the 1960s, when all computers were mainframes, one such machine was called the Datapoint 2000. A label prominently warned about "no user serviceable parts inside." Undeterred, a group of "pesky users" figured out how to make their terminal do work just for them. Years ahead of their time, they saw the future of computing, the PC.

Leadership

Leadership is a job, not a position. The people who work with you are not your people; you are theirs.

Max DePree[6]

Productive organizational change depends on leadership. And leadership is intricately involved with perhaps all aspects of the leader's system. The interrelationships reverberate, amplify, constructively and destructively interfere, create, and destroy many things: ideas, material goods, services, resources, and most importantly, human beings.

Have you thought about the distinction between managing and leading? All leaders are not managers, and all managers are not leaders. Someone once said that managers know how to get up the ladder but leaders know which wall to lean it on.

A leader creates conditions that encourage learning and lead to action. Her personal energy energizes the others. A leader works to remove the organizational barriers to change. She guides decisions and behavior in a manner consistent with the aim of the organization. Sometimes, therefore, leadership means making hard choices and taking tough actions, confronting ignorance and resistance. A leader creates a microenvironment at work that engages the energies of people to work together as a system; the people are committed to optimizing the whole, not just their component part. That microenvironment – that well-led workplace – is perceived as special and more attractive than any other those people might alternatively work in. (I thank Paul Batalden for these views.)

Leaders create a "learning organization," going beyond the notion of the cumulative learning by each individual.[7] A learning organization continually increases what it can do by encouraging growth of individuals and teams; and it continually increases knowledge about what it does, for whom, and how it does it. It tests experience and transforms it into knowledge that all members of the organization can access and act on. In a learning organization, knowledge passes from the individual to the work process; what the organization learns *remains* when individuals leave. Contrast this with organizations that fall into disarray when a key individual leaves.

Leaders are interaction optimizers, they focus on the arrows as well as the boxes in system diagrams. They appreciate how internal competition can be counterproductive for system optimization. They listen, probe, and facilitate many levels of an organizational collective mind – a unit that processes ideas better than might the same number of individuals. They manage conflict in a way that produces learning. They practice principled negotiation, separating people from the problems, focusing on the interests and not the positions, generating a wide variety of options, and establishing mutually agreed upon standards for judgment.[8] Leaders appreciate the diversity of behavioral styles among workers, wisely matching tasks with personality. When difficult behavior disrupts collaborative work, they focus on the behavior rather than the person. Quite importantly, leaders have their followers' *trust*; and they understand the deep commitment this entails. Leaders must be honest and authentic.

Always remember, people can detect authenticity in parts per billion.

Paul Batalden

References

1 Herzberg F. One more time: how do you motivate employees? *Harvard Business Review* 1987:109–20.
2 Csikszentmihalyi M. *Finding flow*. New York: Basic Books, 1997.
3 Kotter JP. *Leading change*. Boston: Harvard Business School Press, 1996.
4 Rogers EM. *Diffusion of innovations*. New York: The Free Press, 1995.
5 Blonder GE. Customers are great innovators. *The New York Times* 1998:Section 3, 12.
6 DePree M. *Leadership jazz*. New York: Dell Trade Paperbacks, 1992.
7 Senge PM. *The fifth discipline*. New York: Doubleday, 1990.
8 Fisher R, Ury W, Patton B. *Getting to yes*. New York: Penguin Books, 1991.

14: The gap is never closed completely

A conclusion is the place where you got tired of thinking.

Arthur Bloch

I wrote this book to "hook" you, to get you caught up in new ways of thinking that can become part of your daily work and enrich it. You now understand that this book offers a paradigm for continually learning from what you do in the NICU – and you now appreciate how this learning differs from what you achieve by reading medical journals. The paradigm is anchored in events and processes; the paradigm embeds outcomes research in the daily work. The approach necessarily entails abandoning many established work habits, for I consider a habit an action elicited independent of system feedback. In contrast, we have looked at ways for our results to inform our subsequent actions.

Where have we arrived?

You are now also equipped to usefully return to one of the central ideas anchoring the entire text. Recall the IOM definition of quality of care from the introduction: "... the degree to which health services for individuals and populations increase the likelihood of desired health outcomes and are consistent with current professional knowledge."[1] By having come this far, you now have knowledge and the tools to:

- understand and build the foundation for continually improving the likelihood of desired outcomes
- begin assessing the operationally defined quality of care in your NICU.

This book is only a starting place; many workers have been travelling for several years along the paths I've highlighted. So although we arrive at the final chapter, we do not conclude. The following sources complement the material we've covered and lead beyond.

Continuous quality improvement

- *Clinical improvement action guide.* Nelson, Eugene C, Batalden, Paul B, and Ryer, Jeanne C, editors; Joint Commission on Accreditation of Healthcare Organizations, 1998.
- *Kaizen (also quality and SPC):* Notice this is a NASA website. Berwick writes about similarities between the work of health care and NASA in the reference cited in Chapter 9. http://www.mijuno.larc.nasa.gov/dfc/kai.html

Statistical computation

- *Stata:* statistical software package for enumerative statistical analysis and limited SPC control charting. http://www.stata.com
- *InStat:* statistical software package oriented for users desiring assistance with choosing and interpreting enumerative statistical tests. Designed for relatively small data sets such as you might generate by local NICU improvement work. http://www.graphpad.com
- *Improvit:* SPC software that creates all the types of control charts discussed in this book. http://www.improvit.com
- *Martindale's statistical calculators:* more than you'll probably ever use or need – an interesting site to explore. http://www.sci.lib.uci.edu/HSG/RefCalculators2A.html

Systems thinking

- *System dynamics in education project:* an MIT site for instructional material. http://www.sysdyn.mit.edu
- *Whole systems:* links and bibliography. http://www.worldtrans.org/whole.html
- *Inspiration software:* useful for process mapping. http://www.inspiration.com

Institute for Healthcare Improvement

- Educational and specific benchmarking programs by leaders in the field, covering varied aspects of continuous quality improvement. http://www.ihi.org

Evidence-based quality improvement in neonatal and perinatal medicine

- The electronic pages of *Pediatrics* for January 1999 (volume 103, number 1) present this special supplement. It is arranged in three sections, "Evidence-based quality improvement, principles and perspectives," "Measurement," and "Case studies." The first section summarizes much of the material presented at length in the present book. In general, the papers are a rich source of illustrative and factual information picking up, I think, where this primer leaves off. http://www.pediatrics.org/cgi/content/full/103/1/202/a

Where to go from here?

Throughout this book I've implicitly assumed that you have evaluative data at hand. Unfortunately, the enormous daily task load of the NICU often does not include explicit and comprehensive processes to capture evaluative data. Assembling such data, as readers well know, represents additional hard work. So how shall we reconcile the substance of this book with the everyday realities of NICU data collection and management? The solution, I think, centers on reducing *muda* associated with NICU data management. Recall our discussion of *muda*, activity without value, from Chapter 4.

We consume resources without adding value when we:

- collect the same patient information more than once
- enter the same information in several places in the medical record and NICU charts
- limit our outcomes research to collecting data about the end-results of our care. This amounts to trying to get a good end-result by inspecting it. (We address this in the chapter on variation. Briefly, outcomes management – inspecting the end-result and trying to change subsequent

outcomes on the basis of that information – is conceptually insufficient. We can improve end-results by using knowledge of factors that are *upstream* in the causal sequence.)

A database software application for the NICU can reduce *muda* and facilitate patient care and research.[2] Readers may already use one.[2] Database software lies at the core of the electronic medical record, the future documentation medium for patient care.[3] Be careful, however, to choose such software by considering factors apart from your first impression of the user interface. Assure yourself that the database software product you are considering reflects a complete data management process – and the process you need. Adopting a database software application means adopting an explicit list of data variables and (typically) a new structural arrangement of the data – a data model. Be careful too, not to confuse entering patient data in a computer and producing a legible note that contains "a lot" of information with effective and efficient data management. The former activities reflect limited and superficial data management aims.

I encourage you to think about what explicit aims you wish to have for the data management process of your NICU. They might include:[4]

- to create an accurate data model; that is, a formal data structure that faithfully represents the work and the results. It is a plan for what data you want and how you structure (link) the data so that you can answer the questions you want to and produce the documentation you need
- over time, to rapidly and inexpensively store and retrieve increasing amounts of patient data, to document what happened and whether it happened well
- to foster decision support
- to protect patient confidentiality
- to improve work flow.

Three core components of the data management process support your effort to evaluate and manage your NICU: an accurate and wide-reaching data model, an effective database software implementation of the model, and specific database administration practices. Indeed, I don't think you can comprehensively evaluate and manage a NICU without them. Unfortunately, the complex interaction between the daily work and how it is represented in database software is far too complicated to discuss adequately in a few pages or even a complete chapter.

I have worked for several years on the data management process of my own NICU, and where I go from here is to write in detail about these things, in a book devoted to managing the data of the NICU. Database software is a central part of the process, so database software ought to be a central part of such a book. I have developed and used point of care NICU database software that creates patient records, automates physician "sign out," and supports NICU evaluation and research questions.[4] I believe that a book about managing the data of the NICU will be especially helpful if it includes this software; to illustrate background principles, demonstrate explicit solutions to key modeling and implementation problems, and to support and accelerate developing your own comprehensive data management process. I hope you'll join me.

References

1 Chassin MR, Galvin RW, National Roundtable on Health Care Quality. The urgent need to improve health care quality. *JAMA* 1998;**280**:1000–5.
2 Slagle TA. Perinatal Information Systems for Quality Improvement: Visions for today. *Pediatrics* 1999;**103**:266–77.
3 Dick RS, Steen EB, Detmer DE, eds. The Computer-based Patient Record: An essential technology for health care. Washington: National Academy Press, 1997:234.
4 Schulman J. NICU Notes: A Palm OS and Windows Database Software Product and Process to Facilitate Patient Care in the Newborn Intensive Care Unit. *Proc AMIA Symp* 2003: in press.

Appendix

This section recaps key ideas – to help you hold on to what you've just read and to facilitate your putting ideas into action

Action is eloquence.

Shakespeare, Coriolanus

There is nothing more frightening than ignorance in action.

Johann Goethe

Appendix: A checklist for thinking about NICU outcomes research

To help generate improvement ideas and put them into action:

1 *Formulate explicit aims for the work of your NICU.* These guide decision-making in general and improvement efforts in particular. Consider the future (the vision for your NICU) along with the immediate aims.

2 *Make complacency intolerable within your organizational culture.* Establish a sense of urgency for improving. Show workers why continuing to do what they do means continuing to get what they get, and why this is unacceptable. Those with influence need to embrace authentically the notion of continuous improvement as a way of being.

3 *Determine what to improve.* Look for *muda.* Look for it everywhere. Ideas may come from processes, results, intermediary indicators, and from people within and external to the NICU. Ask those who work in the unit and those you serve about what could be better (be seriously creative in trying to understand the needs of neonates).

4 *Repeatedly evaluate the relationship between what your customers need and what they get.* Understand how your customers decide about how things are going in the NICU. What do *they* measure? What are *their* judgment criteria? Why do they choose to do it the way they do? Event-specific and process-specific patient (parent) satisfaction surveys tend to yield information capable of driving specific improvement.

5 *Formulate explicit process maps and cause and effect diagrams for the area of concern.* "Type of care" can be a useful organizing concept; disease-specific formulations may entail redundant process information. For example, formulating the process of mechanically ventilating an infant may be more useful than looking at respiratory

failure accompanying bronchopulmonary dysplasia and then on another occasion looking at respiratory failure accompanying surfactant deficiency. Distinguish which steps add value and which do not, and which deal with the core work, the *Gemba*, and which deal with support components. For the sake of improving what is done, depict reality rather than an ideal.

6 *Develop Pareto charts from cause and effect diagrams.* The Pareto principle can focus the change efforts: "20 per cent of the problems will cause 80 per cent of the headaches" for a statistically stable process.

7 *Develop a balanced array of outcome measures from a NICU clinical value compass formulation.*[1] The aim is to attain a multidimensional understanding of the causal pathways that lead to the focus of the improvement effort. The chosen measurement variables should inform your process understanding, leading to improvement in end-results.

8 *When you think you've identified what you will measure, ask yourself: "If we measure these things, will we understand better what is going on here? How so?"* If your answer is vague you will probably find *muda* in what you are doing. Have you aggregated subgroups of data that might be more informative when stratified? Review the suitability of your choice of unit of measurement and unit of analysis.

9 *Carve up the problems into manageable chunks.* Design projects that can be accomplished over a few months and set a time limit for the effort. This approach will help maintain interest and motivation. Also, since you don't know how things will turn out, remember: "Only a fool tests the depth of water with both feet" (African proverb).

10 *Understand the variation of system performance.* Keep the time dimension when you measure processes. Verify that you use explicit and valid decision rules to distinguish signal from noise. Recognize and avoid tampering.

11 *Determine whether the performance results are acceptable.* Work with internal and external benchmarks. Learn from others achieving better results than your facility does.

12 *Identify which measurement variables you think are most important for understanding how your NICU is doing and how to improve it.* Display those variables graphically on one side of one sheet of paper. Monitor performance with

sufficient frequency that you may "change course" when it is meaningful to do so rather than discover something when it is too late to remedy the situation. The ideal is real-time "course correction."

13 *Be inclusive.* In your improvement initiatives, represent all members of the system. Multi-dimensional models better depict reality. Also, people are reluctant to embrace a change when they have not collaborated in its planning.

14 *Remember you are working with people.* Improvement work requires that those involved care about their work. Recognize differences in receptivity to new ideas among staff and adjust your approach accordingly. For a person to work productively and enjoyably, their skills must be appropriately matched to the challenges.

15 *Make all of this a basic and a reiterative part of the daily work.* After all, you are changing your work processes to facilitate continuous learning and informed action.

Reference

1 Nelson EC, Mohr JJ, Batalden PB, Plume SK. Improving health care. Part 1: The clinical value compass. *The Joint Commission Journal on Quality Improvement* 1996;**22**:243–58.

Index

Page numbers in **bold** type refer to figures; those in *italic* refer to tables

SIPOC model 18, **18**
SNAP scores 82
software, statistical 82–3, 99, 137
special cause variation 89, 96, 97
specificity, diagnostic tests 47
standards 1
Stata 99, 137
statistical process control (SPC)
  techniques 66, 95–6, 118,
  119, 137
  control charting *see* control
    charting
  NICU mortality rates 96–9
statistics
  analytic 102–3
  enumerative 102–3
  regression techniques *see*
    regression analysis
  software packages 82–3, 137
    control charting 99
  see also specific packages
study populations 46
subjectivity (in assessment) 19
suppliers *30*, 30–1
Suppliers, Input, Processes, Output
  and Customers (SIPOC) model
  18, **18**
systematic error 46
*System dynamics in education
  project* 137
systems 11–68, 38, 137
  aims 15–17, 60
  boundaries 19–20
  causal webs 22, 57
  complexity 54–6, 113
  data *see* data
  efficiency and waste *see muda*
  "fifth discipline" (Senge) 20–2
  framing 38
  improvement planning 32
  interrelationships 13–14,
    18–19, 27, 57
  linear thinking 13
  operational definitions 14, 15,
    16–17
  optimization 17
  outcomes measurement *see*
    outcomes research
  overview 13–22
  PDCA cycle 57–9, **58**
  people as 17–18, 125–6
  perspectives 4–5, 19–20
  problem identification 73–4
  SIPOC model 18, **18**

thinking 13–22
  see also change; processes;
    quality improvement

tampering, data 84–5, 95–6, 102
  see also control charting
temperature measurement, control
  charting 89–92, *91–2*, **93**
time measurements 81
true negative rate (TNR) 47
true positive rate (TPR) *45*, 45–7

u-charts 118, 119
United States, health care
  spending 5
urinalysis 44–9, *45*, *47*, *48*, *49*

value judgments 78–9
variation
  common cause 88–9, 92, 95
  data 84–94
    characterization 88–9
    measurement 76–8, 79–81
    process characterization 86
    relationships between
      variables 81–3
    understanding 95–104
  NICU services providers 2–3
  random 95
  special cause 89, 96, 97
  see also data
Vermont Oxford Database 109
Vermont Oxford Network
  NIC/Q Project 111
vision 31, 129
  see also change

waste 38–9, 72
  see also muda
Wennberg, John 112–13
Whole systems 137
work
  job satisfaction 126–7, *127*
  of NICU 23–32
  processes *see* processes
  as system 17–18, **18**
  without value *see muda*

XmR charts 90–2, *91–2*, **93**,
  96, 99–101
  data display 118, 119
  individual values (X) 99
  moving range (mR) 90–2,
    93–4, 99